Chapter 1: Why This Book?

If there is one thing I know, it is this: health is something that every person on this planet must hold the most dear. It does not matter what shape, size, or form you are in; it is good health that keeps you going. Think of all those times you ran down the stairs without losing your breath. Or the time you fell sick and recovered quickly. Or the time you had the most exhausting day of your life but didn't succumb to the allure of eternal rest. Your body is beautiful, and it is strong. Or at least, it is born strong. It is made with the ability to recover. And yet, and yet, not all bodies remain in the most optimum health that they could be in.

Health. Now that is a word. When was the last time you stopped for a second to discuss the intricacies of the word? To evaluate how well it resonates with you? Do you feel healthy? But before you say yes, what does that even mean? Do you feel strong when you wake up in the morning? When you go back to sleep? Do you feel like you could take over the world and not have your body crumble under the pressure? Or maybe that's too much. Do you feel like you could run around your block for one hour in the morning and not collapse under the sun? Or maybe that is too specific. Alas, how do you know you are healthy?

Maybe we make it more complicated than it seems. Or rather, the world does. You go out to seek the truth about health, and you come at a crossroads within a crossroads. You step into the world of literature to answer for yourself what it means to have a healthy lifestyle, and suddenly, you are getting shoved into heaps and piles of health-related books that say so much without saying the little that is enough. You read pages and pages and volumes of multiple published authors that talk about multiple aspects of health and a healthy lifestyle, but how do you decide what applies to your customer truth?

In your haze of finding your truth, you get your hands on everything. From cookbooks brimming with elaborate recipes to academic tomes dissecting the intricacies of hypertension management, the shelves are laden with information yet often lack the personal touch and practicality that you may seek. I have been there; you are definitely not alone.

In a sea of dieting books inundated with complex jargon and impractical recipes, it's easy to feel lost and overwhelmed. Like I said, I have been there. I've purchased cookbooks boasting sophisticated dishes that demanded a pantry overhaul and hours of preparation. Yet, in the midst of our busy lives, not everyone has the time, resources, or dedication to commit to such culinary endeavors. And while there are certainly informative works on managing hypertension and smart eating habits, they often drown readers in a deluge of information, leaving them grasping for clarity amidst the flood of details.

If you are nodding along while I write this, you may beg the question: why am I reading this then? And why should you? Why should you choose my book over the myriad others lining the shelves? The answer is rather simple. I won't take you round and round in a circle searching for one perfect way to make you healthy because, if I am honest? There isn't one. There is no one-size-fits-all solution to attain a healthy lifestyle. There are things you need to consider, there are things you need to follow, and there are things you need to be careful of, and some of those things will rightfully stick. And I won't even lie to you by giving you some elaborate definitions of health. For me, health is pretty simple. If you can use your body (and mind) easily, you are healthy. If your body supports you when you feel like giving up, you are healthy. In simple words, if you can trust your physical and mental self to achieve your potential, you are healthy.

Transforming yourself into your own version of a healthy individual comes in many different ways and is found through many different paths taken and tested. And finding this version can be a hard task. You will go after multiple sources, research about multiple findings, read multiple books, and still find yourself confused. Some books will contradict each other. Some books will go into so much details that you will get cross-eyed. And some books will use such complicated language and jargon that you will either question your linguistics or your existence (LOL?). At last, how is it, that one finds this health before losing their own sanity in the seemingly impossible search?

This is how my book, and I with it, offers you something unique. On these pages, you will not find just another rehashing of clinical data or a collection of tantalizing recipes. No, it's a journey through my personal struggles and triumphs, a narrative woven with threads of perseverance, determination, and, ultimately, transformation, which I hope will inspire you on your own healthy lifestyle journey. I find my story to be one of resilience in the face of adversity. It's about battling hypertension and cardiac issues with the guidance of dedicated healthcare professionals and emerging on the other side with newfound vigour and vitality. Once a healthy individual, when I found myself facing adverse health conditions, I was so lost. I was not getting better and I was gaining weight. But then I turned my life around. I found my way back to my own health. After shedding approximately 16 kilograms of fat and overhauling my diet, I found myself liberated from the shackles of hypertension medication. At nearly 61 years old, I look and feel better than ever before, which proves the power of lifestyle choices in shaping our health destiny.

But why share my story, you may wonder? Because amidst all these dense volumes of medical literature and clinical studies, there's a missing voice—the voice of someone who's walked the path, felt the struggles firsthand, and emerged victorious on the other side. Unlike textbooks penned by esteemed professors, my words aren't weighed down by excessive details or detached observations. They're raw, they're real, and they resonate with the heartbeat of experience. This is how my book is made for you: it is meant to connect with you on a personal level. What I write in my book is full of insights I gained from my own journey and experience. Whatever I describe is advised by professionals and confirmed by my own experience. It is not something theoretical, it is shown that it can be done because I am living proof of it. And if it works for me, well, it will most likely work for you too.

Don't just take my word for it—let the pictures speak for themselves. Compare the images captured during my hospital stay in November 2022, when I was at my lowest, with those taken on March 7, 2024, after shedding 8 kilograms of total weight and bidding farewell to hypertension pills. The transformation is undeniable to even a blind eye.

But, of course, it is all about dedication and commitment. If you want to work for something, you must embrace what it demands from you: consistency. There are two sayings that come to my mind here: "If you do nothing, you will get nothing" and "Only those who do nothing do not make mistakes." And what is life if not a series of trial and errors and an ultimate success.

Obesity and hypertension are not just inconveniences; they're silent killers lurking in the shadows, ready to pounce when least expected. But they're not invincible. Through disciplined dieting and a commitment to healthy living, we can reclaim control of our bodies and our lives.

In this book, I invite you to embark on a journey of self-discovery and transformation. Drawing upon my own experiences, as well as the invaluable insights of healthcare professionals, I'll guide you through the maze of weight loss, hypertension management, and healthy living. It's not just about shedding pounds—it's about embracing a lifestyle that nurtures both body and soul, fostering a sense of well-being that radiates from within.

So, if you're ready to take the first step towards a healthier, happier you, join me on this journey. Let's defy the odds, rewrite the narrative, and reclaim our health, one mindful choice at a time. I do not bring you another dieting book. I bring you a roadmap to a better, brighter future. And it all starts with you.

Finally, if you are obese or overweighed you will have at least hypertension issues or diabetics let us say in 80 % of cases. The disease will hit, when you least expect it.. In case of hypertension, which is a silent killer, even if you do not realize that you have hypertension, you just have it. Usually, when you have symptoms like: pain in belly with vomiting, pain in the neck, hands and back, cold sweat, spinning in your head, difficulty in breathing, you just lose consciousness for a second or seconds, fear. These are symptoms before a heart attack. It is obvious that it is too late. In my case, my current 88 year old father when visiting a cardiologist said: "My son, you should check your heart." I did so. Therefore, I skipped a heart attack. Somebody, in my village has hypertension and vomits. In my case, due to changing a cardiologist, cos the first one was useless, and staying with him for four years and having consultation with my dietician I lost 16 kg of fat altogether and after a few months I do not need to ask a doctor for a prescription, cos so far I used 14 pills for hypertension and have still piles of them in a drawer. On the eleventh of April, 2024 while describing it I realize that I have been guided by a Guardian Angel and took it for granted. Yesterday, my father visited my cardiologist, cos his family doctor checked his blood pressure and was too high, so she did prescription for some medication. My father always have too low blood pressure even 97/56, yes even that low. After taking medication from a family doctor it was a little lower. I said to my father: "The medication you have is not known to me, but it must be for beating hypertension, so do not take them. We must go to my cardiologist". So we did so in a few days after making an appointment. You know what my cardiologist said? The same thing, as I told to my father and smiled.   My cardiologist checked my fathers blood pressure, did EKG and scanned his heart. I observed him in action. I only admit that he is good at cardiology. What he said even in doctors jargon was understood to me. My father is 88, there is not everything perfect, but within a norm. I asked if Jardiance and Nonpress could help him for draining veins and removing fibromas. He said No. At his age side-effects could be worse, and the basic principle of the doctor is not to make risky changes. His family doctor gave my father a booklet with spaces to fill with dates and blood pressure. The result was that my cardiologist just looked at medication of his family doctor and results of blood pressure monitoring and after 25 seconds smiled and knew what was going on. What he did more, was to provide excellent check-up of health of my father. He summed it up that my father cannot drive, cannot carry bags of more than 3 kg over a distance of 3 km, yet walking is advisable even 4 km. It was ridiculous as I know that If he lifted with me 25 kg and has been active tremendously, it is not good to switch completely, as it would be worse. I confirm that lifting heavy weights is not applicable any more. Other things are still welcome. Cardiologist does not have to know dieting and exercising rules. I know that my excellent cardiologist telling what my father should not do based his statements on statistics and my father's impaired hearing. My father is 88. Yet, my father's mind is beautiful and fully able. Alas, my cardiologist is excellent operating his modern machines and interpreting intricacies of cardiology.

I wanted to write just a book about healthy lifestyle, yet knowing some medical facts is essential, especially that a good doctor will not knock at your door. Healthy eating and dieting leading to a proper weight is essential, as proper weight eliminates many diseases, so the Key to health is mainly by having a proper weight. What is more, it would be perfect to provide all components your body needs just from proper prepared meals especially healthy meals. Yet, it is not usually possible. We have to rely on supplements, which idealistically should provide or supply what your meals do not provide, even if they are healthy. I do not want to explain further, as it may sound complicated. Through the chapters of this book, you will realize what I mean. I do not want to sound like a published professor, but from my many years of experience of tutoring in London, and methodology, I know one thing. "Marek, keep it simple."

Chapter 2: Let's Talk About My Personal Journey

As I sit down to write this book, I can't help but reflect on the countless dieting books I've encountered over the years. From cookbooks filled with elaborate recipes to guides on managing hypertension, each one promised a solution but often left me feeling overwhelmed and uninspired. It is not that all the books I read felt useless, don't get me wrong. There are many books in the market that hold invaluable information, but all that information just felt like words in a paper. What promised me health did not work; what promised me change didn't even make me motivated. It wasn't until I embarked on my own journey to health that I realized the true value of personal experience and determination.

I have the courage to criticize so called professionals all over the World. You know why? I studied at 3 top universities in Poland. The subjects: English, Maths, Power electronics and Electronics systems of control. I hold master degree, an engineering degree. I attended more than 30 trainings in Poland and in London. One of them: intelligent buildings ending with an exam lasting 5 days in Warsaw and 5 days training of Schneider controllers in Warsaw. One of those two trainings cost   about 10 000 US $ each. The cost of a hotel does not count. I slept in a camping site. An interesting fact: during Schneider training there were about 14 people. 12 of them represented and was sponsored by Schneider. They did not have to pay. 2 others including me paid the whole amount. My sponsor was my 88 year old father. He is 88 now. In a couple of days, there is his birthday. To keep it short, I was a tutor in London registered on www.firsttutors.com, where my frozen profile still is till today. I taught: Maths, ICT and who knows what. I keep my 5 STARS.

So what?

Having all those health issues behind me now and cannot find a professional to prepare a room in my basement for heat-exchanger to use geothermal waters and keeping in mind that his excellency plumber will come in 3 weeks, I have dealt with my health issues and I am doing it by my own. Life? Lucky? Yes!!!!!!!!!

What is more, I have professional tools and machines as those who could come in August do not have. I am serious. I had professionals, really outstanding, and I lent them tools a few months ago. They know me and they are busy. I am their best client.

Why am I writing this?

Those building professionals are like doctors in terms of availability. If you want to go to a doctor while being insured, you have to wait months, years . Fortunately, there are private doctors and here situation is good. You can have your visit arranged within days. In the News, I heart that there are less and less specialist doctors in my country. **Therefore, grab your health into your hands. Start from caring about your health, cos what if a doctor can help you in August 2024 and now it is April, not even A Fool's Day. Sorry, August 2024 is for building professionals. For a doctor, you have to wait months or years.** So, can you convince your ill body to wait so long? Of course not.

Proper weight, healthy eating and some activity will keep your illnesses away, and doctors will be needed in serious cases. Wish you all good health as only money will not buy you health and happiness.

I think that to fully understand my relationship with my personal health, it is important to divide my life into two key timelines: before 2020 and after 2020 (a.k.a. before and after I turned 57). Let's take it from the very beginning, shall we?

Growing up, I never paid much attention to what I ate. Like many others, I indulged in whatever was convenient and satisfying without considering the long-term consequences. Which is expected, I suppose? When you are young, you take too many things for granted, health being one of those things. You just eat whatever nice thing you can get your hands on, not thinking much about what this food could do to you. You look at your surroundings today. The fast-food chains are at every corner, and processed foods are in every store. There is definitely a convenience element involved in the rise and popularity of ready-to-eat meals, but the simple truth is this: if the world is blindly following after something, you are also likely to follow it. If someone asks you for pizza in the early morning, you will probably think, heck, why not? It is tasty, it is convenient, and who has the time to think what is going to do to your body later, right? It is fuel for the body, so just have it, and let's go.

That is the kind of mindset that is not uncommon at all. But when you soon realize what all the junk you have had has done to your body, you experience an epiphany. You finally feel like you have opened your eyes. Like this is the time you need to shift things around for yourself and treat your body as it deserves to be treated. I didn't realize this until much, much later.

Before 57, despite all the non-serious attitude I had towards ingesting good-for-body food, I felt I was very active. I relied on physical activity to maintain my weight and fitness. Running and cycling were my passions, and I spent countless hours exploring the streets of London. I ran a lot, and by running huge distances or riding a bike in London, I was able to lose weight easily, be fit and enjoy life. Seemingly, it did not matter what I ate or how much. I spent a lot of money buying food in London. I used to spend 1100 pounds monthly in 2019 just to buy food. My job was on a playground with autistic children, and I had to keep them safe. I commuted to my workplace by bike, choosing long routes, e.g. from Greenford through parks through Ealing Broadway to Northfields and back after work.

I may add, however, that usually, by the end of the day, while I was sleeping, my muscles used to go cold. It meant that in the morning, my muscles were aching, and it was difficult for me to rise. I had to rise like a paralyzed person and exercise for about at least half an hour to warm my muscles and keep them warm throughout the day. Once my muscles were warm, only then I did not feel the pain. Therefore, commuting to work on the bike and running on the playground was good preparation for a half marathon in Ealing in London hence why I participated and did it.

Because I was physically active, I just needed food in large quantities, and I was slim, fit, and healthy. At that time, I felt no need for a dietician. So before 57, by being active, I did not need to count calories in my food. I know that everybody is different, but my example before 57 addresses young people who, by physical activity, can lose weight, and thus, do not put much focus on healthy eating habits. If all the physical, active work is keeping you fit, who cares about all the unhealthy stuff you are putting in your body?

That reality, however, has a way of catching up to you once you get older. And, as I entered my late fifties, my lifestyle caught up with me. Hypertension became a constant companion, accompanied by cardiac issues that left me feeling helpless and vulnerable. My body began to betray me. Hypertension medication became a necessity, and the looming threat of heart surgery took me by a chokehold, so why wouldn't it?

For four long years, I found myself reliant on hypertension medication. All those medicines were a daily reminder of the toll my unhealthy lifestyle had taken on my body. It was a wake-up call that came with a stark diagnosis from my cardiologist: my artery had become so enlarged that surgery seemed inevitable. The reality of facing heart surgery as a result of these negative health effects was very, very terrifying for me.

The gravity of my situation was further intensified by a doctor's report, which depicted a bleak picture of my heart's efficiency. It was clear that something needed to change, and fast. The solution, my doctor suggested, was to shed excess weight. I had never had to worry about my weight before. When I was younger and active, it was just never a problem. But once you get stuck with obesity, hypertension, and an enlarged aorta, follow in their footsteps. So, losing weight was a daunting prospect, but I knew I had no choice but to confront the challenge head-on.

I refused to let myself surrender to despair. When you are faced with a difficult time, you have two options: you either allow yourself to cry over it, or you do something about it. So I tried to do the latter. With the help of my personal trainer and the unwavering support of my family, I began to reclaim my health one step at a time. Rehabilitation training and dietary consultations became a regular part of my routine as I worked tirelessly to shed excess weight and regain my strength.

Fortunately, with the help of hypertension medication and diligent blood pressure monitoring, I was able to keep my artery from growing any larger. It may seem like a small victory, but when you are facing a war, every small win in combat counts. This development sure gave me hope that change was possible.

As the summer of 2023 approached, I made the decision to seek the guidance of a dietitian. What drew me to her was not just her expertise but also the innovative tools she had at her disposal. Her scale, which worked in tandem with a computer, provided invaluable insights into my body composition, revealing not just my total weight but also the distribution of fluids, grease, and muscle.

Over the course of five months under her guidance, I underwent a remarkable transformation. With her support, I shed 8 kilograms of stubborn fat and replaced it with 8 kilograms of lean muscle mass. What made that possible? The strategic changes I had to make to my diet and lifestyle.

The first step was to confront the harsh reality of my situation. Two hospital photos, taken just over a year apart, served as a sobering reminder of how far I had come. In the first photo, dated November 2022, I looked frail and defeated, a shadow of my former self. But in the second photo, taken on March 7th, 2024, I stood tall and proud, the picture of health and vitality.

The difference was undeniable; it showed my determination and perseverance. But my journey was far from over. With each passing day, I continued to push myself to new heights, embracing a lifestyle of healthy eating and regular exercise.

It may all sound smooth sailing, but I would like to clarify that my road to progress was far from smooth. In the aftermath of my health scare, I found myself grappling with the physical limitations imposed by my condition. Simple tasks like dressing myself became monumental challenges, requiring the assistance of my elderly father. It was a humbling experience, one that underscored the urgency of my journey to health.

When rehabilitation training became a central part of my routine, I was working tirelessly to regain my strength and mobility. My progress was slow, and I faced setbacks more often than not. Even as I regained my footing, there were moments when the enormity of the challenge ahead was so overwhelming that I often felt I was on the verge of losing hope.

I sought guidance from medical professionals, including esteemed professors and dietitians, but their advice often felt disconnected from my own reality. I was doing everything, but I wasn't getting fit. Why? It wasn't until I took matters into my own hands that I began to see real progress. My journey to health began with a simple realization: I had the power to change my own destiny. Armed with determination and a newfound sense of purpose, I set out to transform my diet and reclaim my health.

Through it all, I refused to lose sight of my goal. With each passing day, I pushed myself to new heights, determined to defy the odds stacked against me. On February 16th, 2024, I achieved a major milestone of losing a total of 8 kilograms, which was all due to my unwavering commitment to achieving the health that I deserved. We must not forget that altogether I lost 16 kilograms of fat cos gaining 8 kilograms of muscle is not the same as gaining 8 kilograms of fat. At the beginning of 2023, I was slim coming back from the hospital. Yet, my muscles were not enough. That was the problem. My father had to help me dress, so you see that total weight is misleading. I weighted 100 kg just after leaving hospital. You may think that it is awesome. Yet, it wasn't. At September 2022, I emptied tubes with suntan and gel helping your hair to grow into a toilet. They were German and French. They were excellent, but you have to use such strong chemicals with caution even while exhaling them during proper usage. I got allergic and poisoned, so I just literally got out of my house in chase of fresh air. I ended up on a petrol station and behaved strangely. Within like 1 minute and 30 seconds a police car took me to a hospital 20 kilometers away. At hospital within 10 minutes, I ended up at Toxicology department. They tested me if I took drugs. After 2 weeks I was at intensive care, where I stayed 2 months. It is where two pics were taken by my father. I was also at rheumatology department for 2 weeks. At the beginning of 2023, I weighted 100 kg and needed assistance during dressing up and bathing. Fortunately, I was home and alive. I took a report from hospital, where everything was written. It was described on 6 pages. It looks terrifying, as my blood was exchanged completely. Below my throat there was a hole for feeding. In hospital I was so not aware of what was going on around me, that is why I could not be aware of the gravity of my situation. I am not enumerating what they did to me in hospital, cos it is not important. I know that you realize that at the seventh of April 2024, I can tell that it was a miracle. I am also thankful to Polish police, that they took me instantaneously to a proper hospital and Polish doctors who knew what they were doing. I know that if I waited like 15 to 20 minutes for an ambulance, who knows if I were alive now. Polish police knew to take me to hospital as quickly as possible. All in all, it was a miracle that I am alive. I pray to God thanking for this miracle. I will add that a priest gave me so called the final anointing given to a dying person, who cannot even confess and take a holly sacrament. Therefore, if you managed to get through this, and if you know that it was a miracle, and if you can write it cold-blooded, and if you feel healthy and attractive, you are empowered and you want to share your story. Today, the seventh of April 2024, I met a Lady, who is like 36. She was really attractive like 15 years ago. I was 46 at that time. I was too old for her. I said good morning to her with no reply today. She is /sorry/ ugly now. I feel attractive now.

I am writing all this, cos I think that I received a second chance in life and it is all about healthy lifestyle. Let us compare this to a fight of Sylvester Stallone in "Rocky.....". He was down, there was counting and he rose and won. My story is true. It is not a movie. Today, I feel that I rose and "I am back" /Arnold Schwarzeneger/ and I have my second life.

Yet, it is beginning of 2023. I am finally home with my beloved father. I weight 100 kg. I am slim and weak. My father assists me with bathing and dressing. I could only put on my panties. Across a street, there is a rehabilitation Centre and I was accepted for two weeks for exercises. They lasted like two hours each day. Believe it or not, I could put on a jacket by myself with lots of effort after those two weeks. It was the next step towards progress. It was winter. It was cold. I was not happy to walk outside. I ate a lot, as at the end of staying in hospital, meals there were tasty, but humble. Therefore, I enjoyed eating. Therefore, I lost so many pounds. During summer 2023, I visited "Naturhouse", where worked my dietician. I am not describing in details the progresses and regresses in losing weight, cos it would be boring. Weight may be dynamic especially if you want to lose it. I will tell you that I was about 130 kg during summer 2023. I was slowly instructed about healthy diet and introduced it. Sometimes I lost 1 kg of fat and gained 1kg of fluids. Yet, till the end of December 2023, I lost 8 kg of fat and gained 8 kg of muscles. At the beginning of 2024, I weighted 131.5 kg. Till mid of February 2024, I lost 8 kg of total weight. I weight 123.6 kg even now. It is April 2024. I am still overweight, yet taking into consideration 192 cm of my height and strong figure, I could be happy with my current weight. What counts that from mid of Feb 2024 till April 2024 I did not gain weight. My blood pressure stabilized, and I found myself relying less and less on medication to manage my hypertension. I have still hypertension pills in my drawer, yet I use them so rarely that I do not need to ask for a prescription of my family doctor. After a few months, I used 14 tablets of Lapixen. It proves that I do not need it so much.

My cardiologist is not impressed by my progress or at least does not show emotions. He behaves professionally. He has three rooms for his disposal. There are EKG equipment in one room. He has an equipment for scanning e.g. heart and assess the size of aorta in mm. He has two computers for different purposes. He writes reports about everything precisely and to the point. He prescribes medication and is able to do everything within 10 or 15 minutes. He is a private doctor, which means he must be excellent. He adjusted my medication regimen accordingly. With his guidance, I began a new chapter in my journey to health, armed with the knowledge and determination to succeed. The road ahead is not fraught with challenges. The scenario is simple. Obesity led to hypertension. Hypertension enlarged my aorta. To prevent aorta from further enlarging, my cardiologist said: "Have average blood pressure 120/80". Even being obese and taking hypertension pills, I have kept the same size of aorta for 4 years. With losing each kg of fat, I noticed having more control over my hypertension. I rarely take those pills. We have in mind that my blood pressure must be 120/80 average. Today, the seventh of April 2024 at 5 pm I measured my blood pressure and it is 123/86. It is not bad.

It would be good to achieve 115 kg. I would control my blood pressure even more.

To sum it up:

I have to scan my aorta once a year to be sure that is of the same size.

In order to make scanning aorta once a year a formality, I must

1) **Keep my average blood pressure at 120/80**
2) **Lose another 8 kg to forget completely about beating hypertension pills**

To improve my smooth circulation of blood, I must take Jardiance and Non-press to:

1) **Make my veins and blood circulation "pipes" elastic**

2) **Remove blockages for blood circulation**

3) **Release pressure on aorta due to this magic prescribed medication**

These last medications is necessity while being after maybe 50 due to aging. The similar effect on a smaller scale is consuming Extra Virgin Olive Oil and/or salmon tablets with omega-3. The last thing was confirmed by my dietician.

I am proud to admit that by changing my diet completely, I lost some of the weight I had to lose and I no longer take Lapixen and Telmix Plus religiously. I only take the former when my blood pressure is a little higher, e.g. 127/96. Today, I stand as living proof that change is possible at any age. My journey to health has been marked by setbacks and challenges, but through it all, I have remained steadfast in my commitment to living my best life. This humble booklet is like a journal. On 6th of May 2024 I measured my blood pressure and it was 117/78, which is like an astronomer has-excellent. Over 2 weeks I have not taken any pills beating hypertension. It means that my blood pressure has stabilized. I only lost 8 kg to achieve this and eat healthy foods. I still am overweighed. Does it sound like a motivation to you.

My goal when I began to write this book about a healthy life-style with emphasis on healthy eating, was to impart the insights from my experience to you, dear reader, if you too are facing health issues. Having written it, I must admit that we must not enumerate what to eat, for it will not reflect everybody in every situation. If you live in an area, where climate is cold, would the same kind of food be good for you as for the person living where it is hot? Of course not. If you are a sportsman, skinny and eat a lot, I will not tell you to eat less. If you are young, you need more energy, so you need to eat more.

My motto is simple: Try to eat healthy meals, and introduce healthy customs, as they not only help you to maintain a healthy weight, but whatever you achieve, they will help you to keep it throughout the rest of your life.

As I embrace the next chapter of my journey, I find myself filled with a sense of gratitude and optimism. I may not have all the answers, but I know that by sharing my story, I can inspire others to take control of their own health and well-being. This book is not just a collection of words, it is my promise to you that by perseverance and hard work, you too can reach your health goals like I did. Finally, whatever you want to overcome, you have to know what is wrong, and only then you can know what you have to target. Therefore, proper diagnosis, and then the proper action. More and more people with obesity, or overweight means: heart problems, hypertension, enlarged aorta, diabetes and more. Therefore, my motto to you is:

"Reduce your weight by healthy eating and lifestyles before diseases come to you, when you least expect it."

Chapter 3: Healthy Eating for Life

Before we move any further, let me just tell you one thing: acquiring good eating habits is the only way to live a long and healthy life. And at this point, let me also make it very clear that when I say healthy eating habits, I don't mean dieting. In today's world, it is very easy to confuse the two.

Dieting is usually a very weight-loss-centric prospect. You are on it when you need to lose pounds and then off it once you achieve the goal. The sustainability aspect is not something that one would usually associate with dieting. Just think about all those miracle diets you see on your YouTube and social media. They help you lose weight, and just after you accomplish your weight goals, you find yourself going back to old eating habits, and your previous weight is back. Isn't that just nonsense?

That is why: Acquire good eating habits, make slow but firm steps, and enjoy your life. And more speedy or rigorist changes you make to your diet, the more chances to change or even slow metabolism. Be aware of that.

Having said that, and having in mind new trends targeting to change your metabolism for your benefit e.g. to lose weight, I will not state but just say. The concept of changing metabolism is perfect, but I realize that it is a new thing. Therefore, it just needs further verification.

In our modern world which is so full of fad diets and quick fixes, it's crucial to distinguish between short-term solutions and sustainable lifestyle changes. Once you realize that, you will see how dieting and healthy eating are so different, like two sides of the same coin.

Dieting often connotes restriction, temporary measures, and a focus solely on weight loss. On the other hand, healthy eating is all about a holistic approach to nourishment. It considers not only physical health but also mental and emotional well-being. It's about forming habits that promote vitality, longevity, and overall quality of life. Does eating healthy promote weight loss? It could or it could not because the weight loss game is all about the hide-and-seek between calories in and calories out. But does healthy eating promote your overall physical well-being in the long run? Absolutely yes.

In this chapter, we will discuss many different aspects of healthy eating habits, including some of my own tried and tested recipes and meals that can bring you the nourishment you need. But before that, there are some principles that make the essence of healthy eating, and hence, you should know.

Principles of Healthy Eating:

1. Variety: Incorporate a diverse range of foods in your everyday palate and plates to ensure your body receives many different nutrients from many different sources. Why? Because this helps promote optimal health and vitality. Embrace fruits, vegetables, whole grains, lean proteins, and healthy fats to create a balanced plate.

2. Moderation: Enjoy all the healthy foods you like. The catch? Do so in moderation. Why? Because it allows for flexibility and prevents feelings of deprivation. Focus on portion control and mindful consumption.

3. Nutrient Density: Prioritize foods rich in essential nutrients, such as vitamins, minerals, fibre, and antioxidants. Why? Because these nutrient-dense options fuel the body, support immunity, and enhance overall well-being.

4. Balance: Strive for balance in every meal, incorporating a combination of macronutrients (carbohydrates, protein, and fat) to sustain energy levels and promote satiety. Why? Because life is all about balance.

The above principles might have helped you understand what healthy eating is actually about, but for anyone on a health-related journey, finding clear paths of action is so difficult. I know. I say that as someone who has struggled with finding precise directions on my journey as well. If it is beginning to overwhelm you, stop for a second. I need you to breathe and close your eyes; it is okay.

You can't route learn your way through a healthy lifestyle. Exploring healthy eating habits and then sticking with ones you can follow consistently is what makes them sustainable. You have nothing to worry about. Right now, it's all about shifting focus and finding your resolve to start. The rest of the things will flow much naturally and easily.

Let's break down a few tips and tricks you can follow to adopt a healthy diet and a healthier lifestyle.

Healthy Eating for a Healthy Life: A Check-List

Guide:

1. Mindful Eating: Cultivate awareness and presence during meals. Savor each bite and pay attention to hunger and fullness clues. Avoid distractions such as screens or multitasking, because once you lose focus while eating, it is so easy to overeat in a haze. Allow yourself to fully engage with the sensory experience of eating.

2. Cooking at Home: Take control of your food choices by preparing meals at home whenever possible. This empowers you to select wholesome ingredients, experiment with flavours, and tailor dishes to meet your nutritional needs.

    Cooking at home vs meals at certain college in London

    "There is no comparison. Those meals and drinks at that college are totally unacceptable. Unhealthy. Yet, there were fountains with filtered water and even cups for one usage free of charge.

3. Hydration: Stay adequately hydrated throughout the day by drinking water and other hydrating beverages. Go for water-

rich foods such as fruits and vegetables to boost hydration levels and support overall health.

4. Consistency: Establishing consistent eating patterns fosters stability and promotes sustainable habits. Aim for regular mealtimes to maintain steady energy levels and prevent overeating.

Tips:

1. Buy a smartwatch or a smart-phone or both especially if they cooperate with each other.

They can do the following things:

a. monitoring number of steps you take to control your daily walking target so that you can maintain a certain amount of physical activity, which would stimulate and help you to stay fit.

b. measuring the amount of oxygen in your blood. If it is 90, it is OK. If you are somewhere in the open air or have your window open, you may try to take deep breath, hold it for a second, and breathe out. After a while, in my example, I can reach even 95. According to my logic, if there is more oxygen in your blood, you are speeding digestion, a good thing for remaining healthy.

c. measuring blood pressure. Remember: 140/90 is the borderline. This function is now in many smartwatches, but I personally use a traditional blood pressure monitor for the upper arm. My cardiologist also recommends it, so I guess you should go with the option that is more convenient for you and the last not least provide correct info.

2. Modify your meal timings

If you decide to eat 3 or 4 times a day, make sure to eat at precise times. It means no eating anything between meals. No snacks between meals.

3. Try to eat just a little less than when you feel like you are full

The thing is, even if you eat a little less than the feeling that you are full, after 20 or 30 minutes of finishing your meal, you will feel full.

This is exactly why you feel like you are bursting at the seams a few while after you eat a large, large, meal.

4. Take your time when chewing your food

This is also connected to the previous point in a way. Because if you eat slowly, you will probably eat less than if you eat large amounts of food quickly.

5. Instead of thinking about food in your free time, try to keep your mind busy and focused on any other task.

It is logical, and it works. If you are busy with something, time flies. And when you are not, the idea of food becomes a hobby. "Hmmm, I am bored. Why don't I grab that one slice of leftover pizza in the fridge. Or snack on my chocolate bar I didn't have the chance to finish." You see? But when you divert your attention, you help yourself to stay away from food between meals. On the other hand, when you divert attention while eating, you do not know that you are eating. That is why, you are eating a lot.

6. Drink water 15-30 minutes before your meal

This is simple: drinking water before your meal decreases your appetite, saving you from stuffing your face- because that is definitely NOT a healthy way of eating.

7. Avoid moments of being hungry for too long

If, under any circumstances, you let yourself remain hungry, it will eventually only lead to one thing: you will end up overeating. You will eat a few times more than usual, and again, that is far from healthy.

8. Stay physically active according to your age and all other things.

It is possible to lose weight without exercising, although that does make it easier to reach your weight goals. But we are not just talking about weight loss here. We are talking about a sustainable healthy lifestyle, something that continuous physical stimulation makes it easier for you to achieve.

9. Let your diet be balanced

Let me be real: following a balanced diet is easier said than done. Realistically, it might not even be as possible as the fitness influencers online may help you believe. Yet, still, it is something that should be aimed at. It is necessary to provide your body with all the nutrients and components it needs to promote its well-being. It is not just about energy: vitamins, minerals, and all other nutrients help us thrive in life.

10. Drink proper amounts of water

Water is far more important than food.

11. Limit the consumption of red meat

Research suggests that a high intake of red meat, particularly processed varieties, may increase the risk of cardiovascular disease, certain cancers, and type 2 diabetes.

12. Avoid sweets, chocolate, sugar, salt, and alcohol

High intake of sweets and sugary foods can lead to weight gain, insulin resistance, and increased risk of chronic diseases like diabetes and heart disease.

Excessive salt intake can elevate blood pressure and contribute to cardiovascular issues.

Alcohol, when consumed in excess, can impair liver function, disrupt sleep patterns, and increase the risk of addiction and various health problems.

Considering the health risks associated with all these, it's advisable to consume them in moderation and prioritize nutrient-dense foods to support overall well-being.

13. Try to avoid butter and margarine

It's better to steer clear of both butter and margarine due to their high saturated fat content and potential health risks. You can buy "Humus" as an alternative to butter and margarine.

I want to add that I am quite aware of what I write. I am not a coward. I must add that I pay attention to consistency and details. I read everything over and over again and again. I am correcting certain sentences and add new information. I will not write that this book is for entertainment purposes only as some writers about Mediterranean diet. It would be not right, as my goal is healthy lifestyle and health issues. There is no place here for jokes and tricks. I am not afraid of legal cases. Whatever is written here was proposed by professionals and tested on me or even verified by me. I was like a laboratory mouse, which like in case of ending up in hospital and challenged with all those things, there was no way back. I ended up in hospital not due to mistakes at dieting or healthy life-style. It was explained somewhere else in this book. Sometimes, if you are half way in one direction, coming back or attacking and moving on does not make any difference. In my journey, I am relieved now. I cooperate with the best of the best. My current cardiologist is my second one and I go to him once a year to scan my aorta. It is enlarged, yet it must keep its size. /Once, my family doctor listened to my heart beats, and said "I hear noise, you must go to a cardiologist." I repeated it to my cardiologist and commented: "If I have my aorta enlarged, it is normal." My cardiologist smiled back. My dietician is the same, as she is perfect. She is young and from the beginning of this year, she runs her own dietician business. For the last two weeks, she has begun so popular that this week I had a choice to visit her on Wens in the afternoon or tomorrow at six pm. She is busy.

Chapter 4: Healthy Meal Prep with Yours Truly

Your journey on healthy eating is going to be all about the fundamental shift from even eating processed products even fast foods /rubbish food/ to nourishing your bodies with wholesome, nutrient-dense foods. While dieting is mostly about counting calories, healthy eating is more about exploring the significance of quality over quantity and the profound impact it has on overall well-being.

To aid in this transition, I have prepared some practical examples of preparing meal items that not only support weight loss but also promote optimal health. I have included these in my book because they worked for me and millions of others worldwide, and I hope they work for you, too.

First things first, water!

Drinking water is fundamental! I have talked about staying hydrated, and I will say it again. Water is so important, and while you may have not thought about this before, there are ways to prepare water as well.

The easiest way is to buy bottled water.

If you want to use tap water, you have to have a jar with a filter to intake the proper quality of water. A filter has to be replaced according to the manufacturer's instructions. In Westfield Shepard Bush Shopping Centre, there is a whole fountain with cooled, filtered water of fantastic quality.

I used to filter water, but for me personally, it did not taste right. Therefore, I prefer to boil water and let it cool. I use a designated glass jar to keep such water.

Yet, I do not do it anymore even if it is not bad. For like one year, I have been drinking just still mineral water from a shop.

Intaking only water for all days can feel boring, no?   While reading this piece about water, I want to emphasize sth. ,if you want to stay healthy. I buy water in 1.5 litre plastic bottles. I trust that plastic bottles nowadays are different that those like 20 years ago, yet be safe and do not expose plastic bottles to sunlight. I exchange SMS with my dietitian and she emphasises to drink 3 litters of water daily. Tea and other soft drinks do not count. Actually I do not drink nothing apart from mineral water and tea. 3 litres for a big man like me. **With**

aging you do not want to drink water so much, but your body needs it.

From time to time, I buy food in one particular good store. Because I bought food for nearly 100 US $, they asked me if I wanted a pack of coke for 25 cents. I replied: "No, thank you".

During cold days, try some tea!

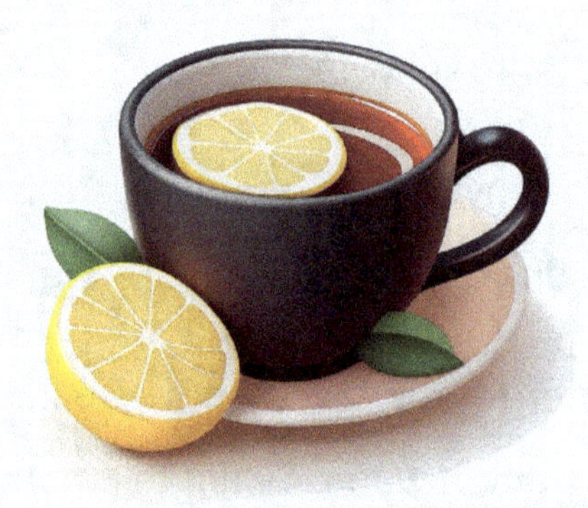

I love black tea and grey tea.

To properly prepare a cup of tea, boil water, pour some hot water into a cup to warm it, empty the cup, and then pour hot water into the cup; add one teaspoon of tea and two teaspoons of natural sweetener. Maybe even a slice of lemon later. Grey tea should not be served with any other things.

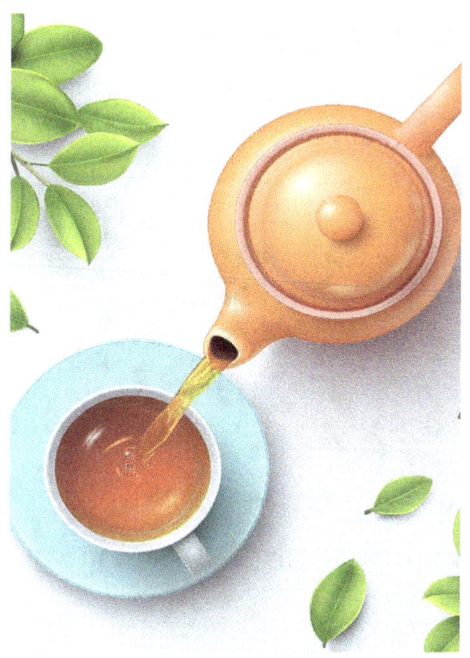

This is a jar for brewing tea!

Warm the jar with hot water and empty the jar. You put tea from the top and pour hot water from the top. If you let it brew for 5 minutes, then you can have delicious tea.

It is a good idea to visit a tea shop and get to know various kinds of tea, ranging from black tea and grey tea to herbal tea. Some herbal teas are for stimulating digestion, so if you want to lose weight, you should know the whole approach to reach your goal. Of course, you should always know the limits, as exaggeration can lead to some digestive sensations.

An example of breakfast or supper

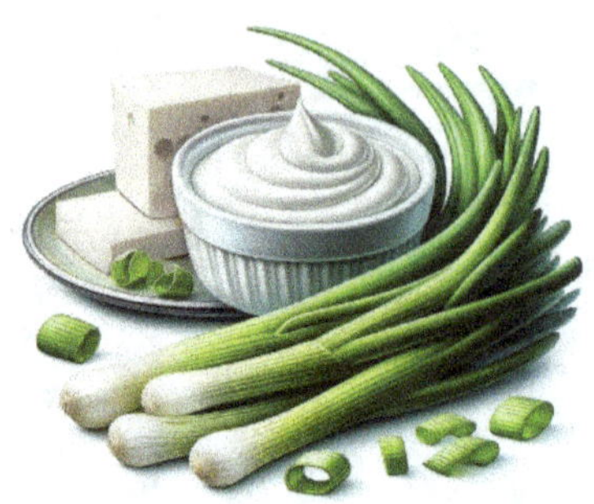

Above, we see an open package of cream from the top. In the middle, that is an onion, and at the bottom, there is white cheese.

If you take a bowl, put the content of white cheese inside, cream and chopped onion, then add spices like pepper and so on. It is up to you. Then, mix it together. You will have a tasty white cheese. It will come with slices of bread. No margarine and no butter. As an alternative to butter or margarine, I propose HUMUS.

It will come well with black tea with Erythritol /natural sweetener/

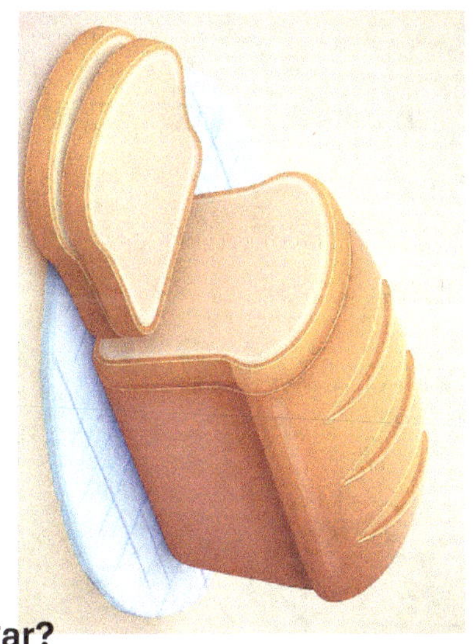

What about sugar?

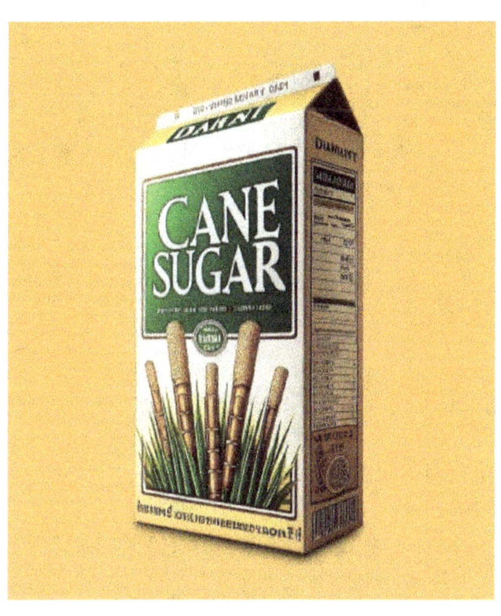

For more than ten years, I had used this cane sugar. From my sources, this sugar is healthier. Yet, sugar is caloric. Sugar contributes to damaging teeth and is wonderful to multiply bad bacteria in your stomach.

Yet, if you want to lose weight, buy natural sweeteners containing 0 calories.

An example of a dinner

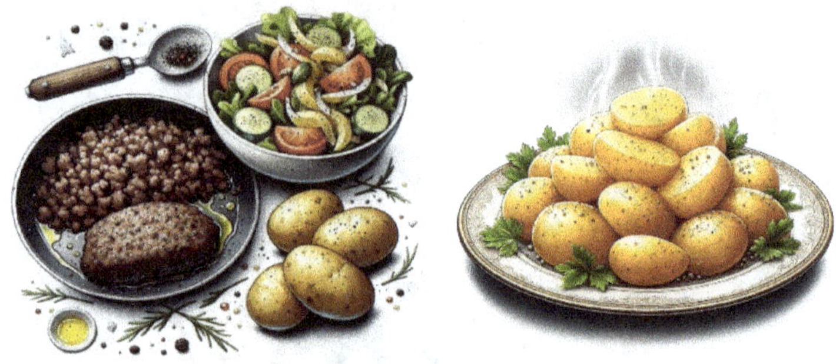

On the right-hand side, you have boiled potatoes. You can add just a little oil from the pan where these two pieces of minced meat are fried. Just a bit of pepper and other spices. I would suggest adding another plate with an Italian salad sprinkled with olive oil and a little lemon squeeze.

But what about healthy oils when cooking a meal?

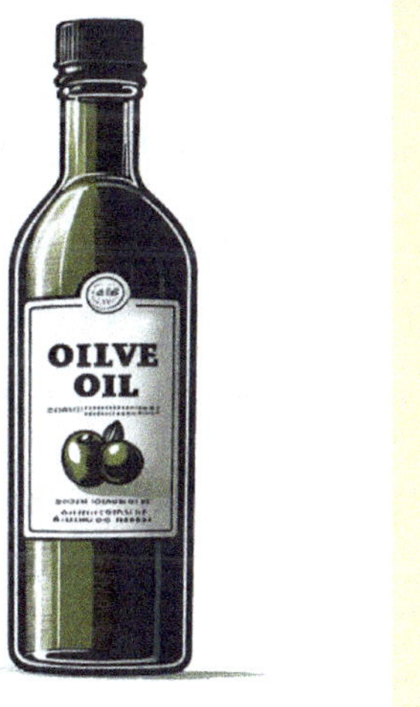
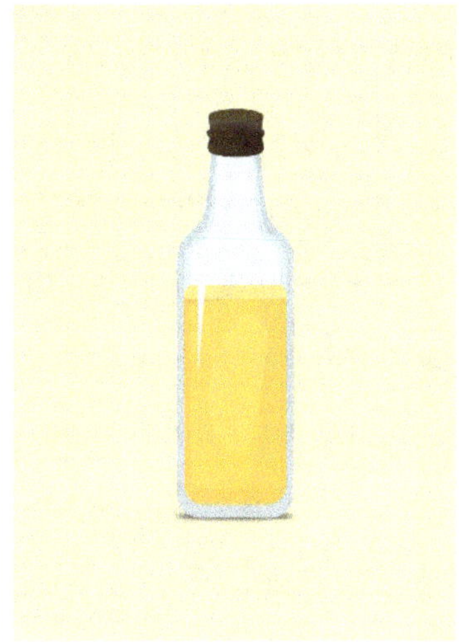

We have Extra Virgin Olive Oil, and ordinary oil for frying.

The first one I use for salads and the second one for frying items. If you used olive oil for frying, the oil you are using would be more expensive than what you are frying. Be economical!

I strongly recommend Extra Virgin Olive Oil for salads. It is excellent due to Omega-3 component.

I will only add that I have read a large article about this oil enumerating benefits to our health by consuming it.

I do not want to paraphrase that article, as I want to keep everything as simple as it is possible. I was just stunned by what they wrote. It is a good natural medication from Mother Nature. Above I am frying minced chops using a thick pan. Why? It takes more time for the pan to take heat than give it back to what you are frying. It gives you control. If your meal is ready and the pan is still hot, you can take your meal from the pan. Also, if your meal is nearly ready, you take the pan out of the stove and accumulated heat in the pan will finish frying. You also avoid sticking the food to the pan and limit amount of the oil you are frying with, cos e.g. this particular pan is thick for the reason. You could fry even without oil. Yet, in reality I add a little oil.

How to prepare minced meat chops?

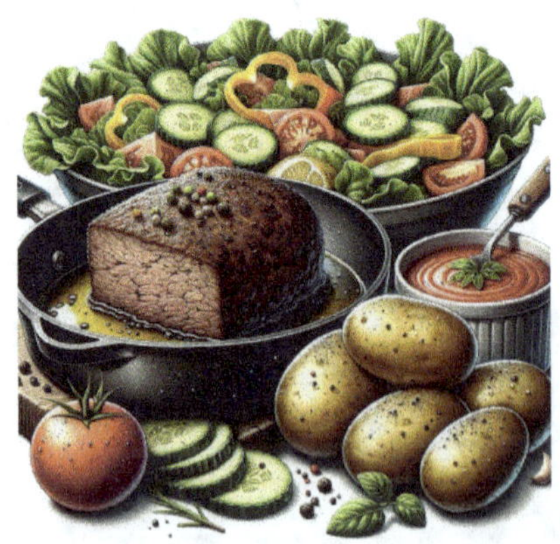

Components: Fresh minced meat, chopped onion, roll soaked with water, one egg, and spices.

Put them inside the bowl and mix together.

With washed hands, form thin chops and cover them with flour. Put them in a hot frying pan with some oil on the bottom.

Alternatively, you can fry a fish in such a pan.

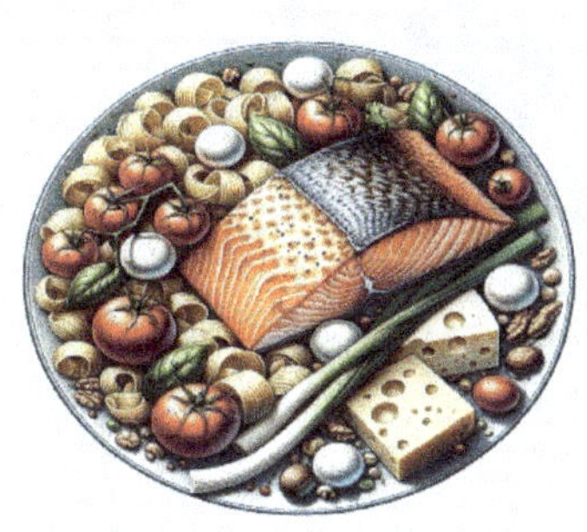

If you have a fresh fish, you have to remove what is inside properly and remove eyes. You have to scrub with a knife the fish to remove sliperry covering of a fish. Clean the fish with water. Wait till the water just disappears a little bit. Leave the fish head untouched and cover the fish with flour. Deep fry so that the skin of the fish would be hard. Not cutting the head off of the fish before frying keeps the fish in one piece.

To be real, fish is an even better option because it is healthier.

Another alternative for dinner on a sunny day

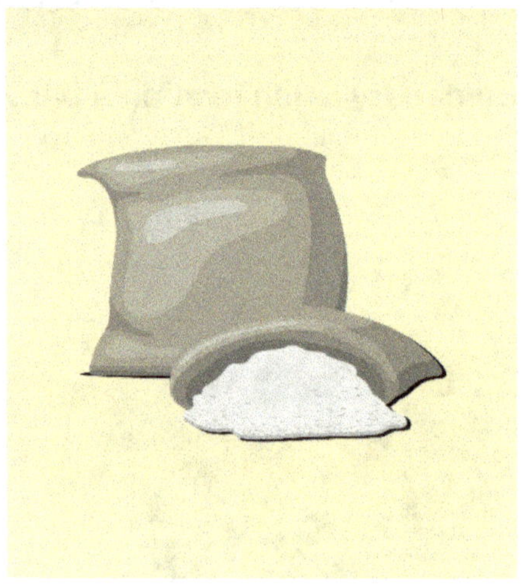

That is rice. You can buy a package of rice in small bags. You boil such rice in hot water for about 10 minutes. Check the instructions on the package.

You will need yoghurt and strawberries to make it healthier and tastier. Just put them on the top of rice.

Another dinner alternative for a hot day

Imagine a complete dinner I sometimes have during a hot day.

It consists of boiled potatoes, fried fish, boiled green beans and chopped dill on the top of potatoes. It was my second meal during a hot day. This meal stops you from being hungry.

I bought the frozen fish from a shop, and since it was clean, it only needed frying. This made for a quick meal prep, but a better alternative is to buy fresh fish from Fish Monger. Though, you will have to spend more time preparing it. Green Beans and potatoes need boiling.

Include some dill in your diet.

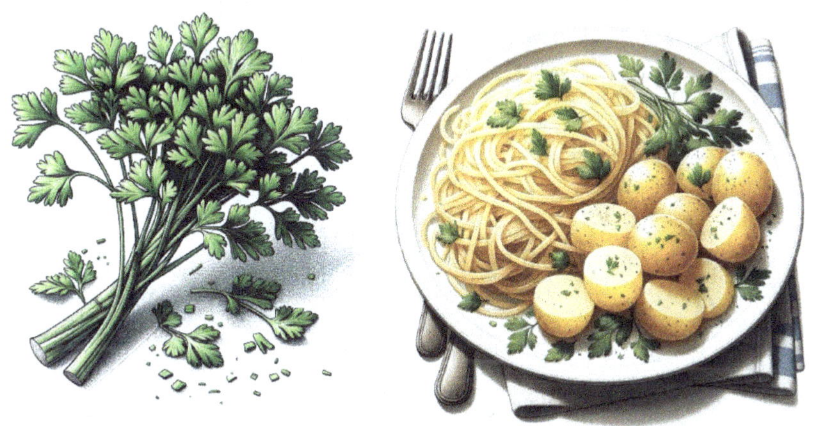

Before putting it on the potatoes, you just need to wash it and chop it. Such a component eaten with potatoes helps you digest the whole meal better.

Isotonic drink

Isotonic drinks do not contain sugar. Sugar is replaced with artificial sweeteners- yet be sure that you are not allergic to it. The concept of replacing sugar is to eliminate excessive calories.

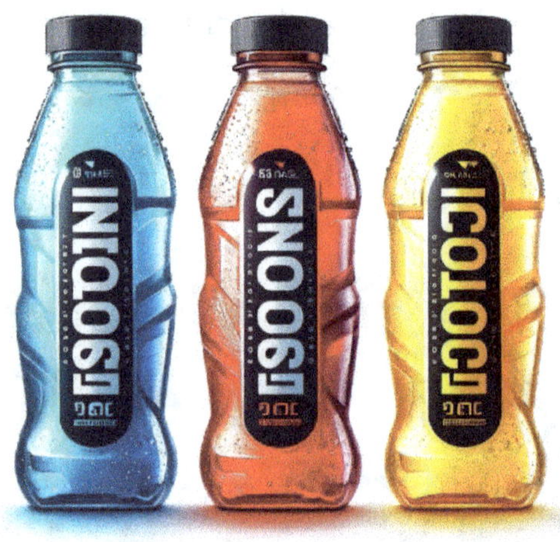

Isotonic drinks are for sportsmen or sportswomen, as they contain minerals and other components you lose while sweating. They are more important to you than sugar. This drink can be useful to you, as during a hot day you are sweating as well. On hot days, I usually skipped my tea for this soft drink, but for the last year I have been drinking just still mineral water on hot days.

Salads are of the utmost importance!

This salad is fantastic for the meal. You can see five baby tomatoes, which can be replaced by ordinary tomatoes, yet these are just awesome. This salad, apart from tomatoes, is sold foiled and comes from Italy or Spain. I noticed in London that artificial wall climbers bought this salad. You just add a little bit of olive oil and soya sauce, and it tastes so delicious.

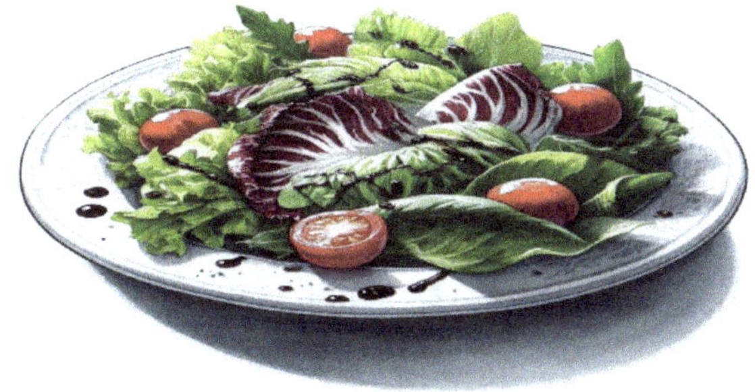

Salads are not a meal on their own, though, so make sure you eat it with more concrete food.

To complement a healthy diet, we cannot neglect vegetable juice!

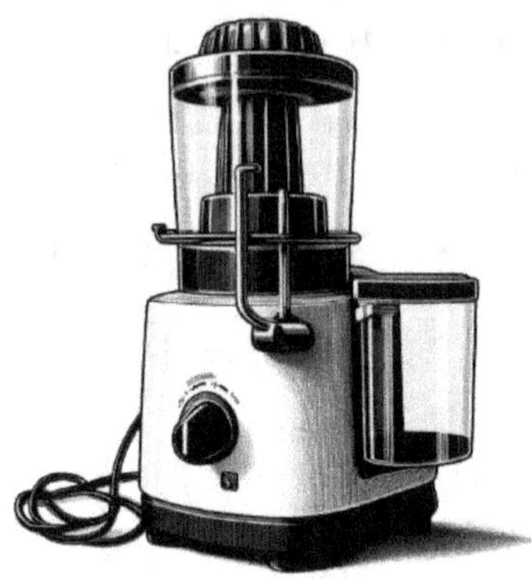

This is a cheap juicer I used, which actually does the job. The remaining vegetables, after extracting juice from them, are dry, so you can use this machine, cos dry vegetables proves that the machine is efficient.

If you put carrots, apples, and celery through the top, with the machine plugged in, of course, you will receive juice from the right side. The juice is tremendously healthy, and I highly recommend it. This cheap juicer looks like it has been working for many years, and that is because it has. I bet that you had an impression that the top of this machine and a small container on the left side are dirty. You are wrong. Vegetables have reacted with the plastic for many years, and you cannot remove it. Anyway, it proves the point that this machine has been used a lot, and I love it. At least, I know what I am describing.

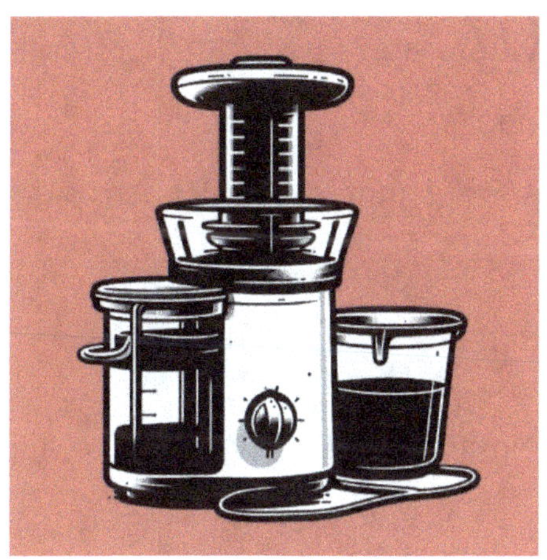

This is a slow juicer. It looks elegant, and the difference from the previous machine is that it extracts juice slowly. It would be better to apply more pressure to receive juice than to use a quickly rotating motor. The result is better quality juice. This machine also makes salads, which may come in handy for families with children.

I recommend a slow juicer, yet I encourage you to eat raw apples as you eat fibre as well, which makes you feel full quicker, so you will not be hungry. My dietician explained it to me, so I must admit that she was correct.

My compromise would be:

- Use slow juicer to enjoy benefits of celery and carrots, cos it looks difficult to eat whole carrots and celery

- Eat e.g. whole apples for fibre preferably one fruit for second meal and supper. First meal contains soya soup with wonderful ingredients and a pear and dinner is served with salad, so that is why you do not need an apple with them.

- Supper should be around 7 pm. One apple with supper is OK. I remember that you should not eat fruits for supper, yet I meant larger quantities. "One apple a day keeps your doctor away"- as it contains some minerals and vitamins. Apple also stimulates digestion and contains fibre to make you feel full.

- After 7 pm drink only water till 9 pm.

I know that for those who work on night shifts e.g. what I mentioned above does not apply in reference for timing.

Eating fruits is also a good practice.

In a certain book, somebody wrote that different colours of fruits are correlated with different vitamins they have. Regardless of how true that is, there is no doubt that fruits are healthy and natural sources of fuel for your body. Therefore, try to eat fruits every day.

However, fruits contain sugar, so eating them in the evening is not a good idea.

If you are thinking: Do they even work?

As I've mentioned before, my book is all about healthy eating and lifestyle, with a particular focus on weight loss for those grappling with overweight issues and striving to maintain a wholesome lifestyle. Drawing from my own journey, which has involved grappling with a bit of obesity and accompanying health concerns, I've poured my genuine experiences into the pages of this book.

Being 61, I find myself still on a quest to shed a few extra pounds. While I might not fare too poorly compared to others, there's still a bit more weight I aim to lose to feel truly content with my health. Despite the challenges posed by the pandemic and the prolonged periods of being cooped up indoors, I've managed to make some headway in my weight loss journey. This, to me, proves the efficacy of the dietary principles I advocate for in my book.

Considering the ever-important factor of budget, I must mention my living situation—I reside with my father, who's 88. We share discussions about our dietary choices, and despite our proximity to the mountains, we haven't forsaken fish from our meals, owing to its undeniable nutritional value. Opting for meat, which is nutritious has been a recent shift in our household. A while back, my father prepared some minced meat chops that were not only delicious but also left me feeling satisfyingly full. Consequently, we've said goodbye to sausages, ham, and other processed meats, much to our wallets' delight. A recent trip to the supermarket was an eye-opener to the rising prices of food items, making the economic aspect of our dietary choices all the more valuable.

It's worth noting that I've dabbled in various weight loss products over time, only to find them falling short of their promises. This underscores a simple truth: our bodies metabolise what we eat, and an excess of calories invariably translates to stored fat. While it's tempting to entertain the notion of a perfectly balanced diet leading to impressive results, the reality comes at its own pace and form.

Hence, your healthy lifestyle will all be about adopting a healthy eating regimen tailored to your individual needs. Understanding our bodies' signals and calibrating our intake accordingly is key. However, diet alone isn't sufficient. Physical activity is equally indispensable—an observation that has been promoted for ages. You cannot discount the favours of physical activities like exercise; you just can't. What is more, physical activity is good for our health even if we have a perfect weight!!!!!!!!!!!!

In essence, the meals detailed within this booklet are designed to be both nutritious and economical and without any unnecessary additives for simplicity and wholesomeness. While convenience foods may seem tempting, they often come at a premium cost. Therefore, the best and healthy course of action would be to go for the homemade meals, and enjoy their nutritional value in the cozy confines of one's humble abode.

Chapter 5: Losing Weight, the Healthy Way I

From summer 2023 till the end of December 2023 I lost 8 kilograms of fat and gained 8 kilograms of muscles. Therefore from summer 2023 till mid Feb 2024 I lost 16 kilograms of fat. It should be emphasized that I lost 16 kg of fat. Gaining 8 kg of muscles was welcome for me to control my body and be able to dress independently. Focusing on the total weight only is completely unprofessional. You cannot just think about biceps and triceps, breast muscle and so on. Our body contains over 600 muscles. Around our spine there are lots of them to protect and cooperate with it. That is why, do not focus on the total weight only.

At the beginning of January 2024, I weighed 131.5 kilograms. As you can imagine, I was at a loss for what could be done. Yet, due to cooperation with my dietician with whom I exchange SMS I learnt a lot about dieting and healthy eating, so till the mid of Feb 2024 I knew what to do to lose weight, yet I did not expect the final result to be that good. Obesity and hypertension had become my constant companions, and I realized that to combat both, I needed to focus on one thing alone: losing weight. But when I say losing weight, I don't mean doing everything I can to shed some pounds without any concern for my well-being: that is not how sustainable weight loss works. Your dieting and healthy eating should go hand in hand; otherwise, there is literally no point in the lower number you see on a scale. A lower weight does not always mean you are healthy, for you can't be healthy unless you achieve that through a healthy lifestyle.

Dieting forms the cornerstone of any weight loss journey, and mine was no different. However, the key lies not in drastic measures or deprivation but in adopting sustainable lifestyle changes. Instead of resorting to extreme calorie restrictions or crash diets, you need to focus on following a balanced eating plan rich in whole foods. Remember, sustainable weight loss is a marathon, not a sprint. And ironically enough, I realize that I have experience in both. Fun fact: I ran half a marathon in Ealing in London, so I know the kind of patience and determination that is needed. And like a marathon, losing weight requires the same level of patience, determination, and commitment to see things through. Like every kilometer covered is a measure of progress in a marathon, every kilogram lost is in weight loss. With every kilogram you lose, that becomes your motivation to keep on going. The key is: Don't Give Up! With every kilogram you lose, your control over hypertension improves. Beating hypertension is a process. It is not that after losing 18 kilograms of fat, I regained the full control over eliminating hypertension. I realize that I noticed that my problems with hypertension were diminishing, yet at that time I did not know why. A few years ago, my blood pressure after a short sprint could be 170/120 for a moment, but I did not dare to tell it to my cardiologist. I took Lapixen to lower my blood pressure at that time. Within 20 minutes after taking it, my blood pressure stabilized. Yet, on one hand if you have to lower your blood pressure, cos it goes crazy, it is good to have Lapixen. On the other hand, it is better to have average blood pressure 120/80 due to proper weight and do not have to take Lapixen. My mind is aware that playing hide and seek with hypertension by monitoring blood pressure and applying Lapixen is necessity not to have .... , but roller-coaster of blood pressure is not what I recommend. At present, knowing that proper weight stabilizes blood pressure I strongly advise to lose weight to avoid hypertension, enlarged aorta, diabetics and more.

Dieting often carries connotations of strict rules, deprivation, and temporary measures. However, a sustainable approach to dieting involves shifting this mindset to one of nourishment, balance, and long-term habits. It took me about half a year to shift my mindset. That is why it took me half a year to lose 8 kilograms of fat, and another 8 kilograms were lost during one month and a half, cos my mind was taught all those tricks and I knew what to do to lose weight. I have prepared a short guide for you to understand how you can adopt a healthier and sustainable approach to dieting:

1. Focus on Whole Foods: Instead of just focusing on calorie counting or restrictive meal plans, prioritize whole, minimally processed foods at the beginning. These include fruits, vegetables, whole grains, lean proteins, and healthy fats. Whole foods provide essential nutrients while also keeping you full, which makes it easier to manage hunger and cravings.

2. Embrace Moderation: Despite eating healthy food, you have to embrace moderation. A good approach is to practice portion control and mindful eating.

3. Listen to Your Body: Pay attention to hunger and fullness clues. What does that mean? Eat when you're hungry and stop when you're satisfied. Avoid eating out of boredom, stress, or

emotion, and learn to distinguish between physical hunger and emotional cravings. By tuning into your body's signals, you can develop a healthier relationship with food and prevent overeating. Finally, feeling full comes after like half an hour after finishing eating. Therefore, you should eat slowly and finish not feeling completely full.

4. Make Gradual Changes: Sustainable weight loss is not about making drastic changes overnight but rather about implementing small, manageable adjustments over time. Start by incorporating one healthy habit at a time, such as adding an extra serving of vegetables to your meals or swapping sugary beverages for water. Gradually build upon these changes as they become a part of your daily routine.

5. Practice Mindful Eating: Mindful eating involves being present and aware of your food choices, eating slowly, and savoring each bite. By practicing mindfulness during meals, you can better recognize hunger and fullness clues, appreciate the flavors and textures of your food, and develop a greater sense of satisfaction from your meals. Eating less and eating healthy food will sharpen your taste-buds in your mouth esp. if you do not smoke.

6. Stay Consistent: Consistency is key to long-term success in any weight loss journey. Instead of viewing dieting as a short-term fix, commit to making sustainable lifestyle changes that you can maintain over the long haul. Set realistic goals, track' your progress, and stay accountable by reaching out for support from friends, family, or a health professional.

I am saying this from my own personal experience: by embracing dieting as a sustainable approach focused on whole foods, moderation, and mindful eating, you can achieve lasting weight loss results while nourishing your body and having a healthier relationship with food. Remember, the journey to better health is not a sprint but a marathon, and by adopting sustainable habits, you'll surely cross every kilometer of your running track and see progress in shedding extra kilograms.

My Own Daily Diet

My dietician suggested the following diet for me after assessing my kilocalories needs as being 2400. If we assume that I have minimal daily activity, my body needed 2400 kcalories just to maintain my weight, which was 131.5 kg. Therefore, if I wanted to lose weight, I had to provide not 2400 kcalories daily by eating my meals, as 2400 calories were needed just to maintain 131.5 kg. This means that I had to take away 400 kcalories from 2400 kcalories, which is 2000 kcalories, to reduce my weight to below 131.5 kilograms. An example diet that I provide below includes 2000 kcalories, and due to such an example diet, I was able to have 123.6 kg on the 22nd of February, 2024. What is more, after achieving 123.6 kg I have to correct my kcalorie intake from 2400 to let us say 2200. After taking away 400 kcalories from 2200, we have 1800 kcalories to lose more starting from 123.6 kg.

Stay Hydrated, but also:

It is a good idea to start your day with two glasses of warm water, boiled about 15 to 20 minutes before your first meal.

First Meal

- Boil one glass of soya drink or milk and one glass of water with 30 grams of oat flakes.
- Add sliced washed pear, 30 grams of cashew nuts, a teaspoon of honey, and a little bit of cinnamon.
- Include 150 grams of Icelandic yogurt.

This first meal is good to be eaten on a daily basis. It is healthy, low-calorie, and gives you the feeling of being full.

Second Meal

- Take three slices of bread and 30 grams of humus (as an alternative to butter or margarine). While having 123.6 kg, my dietician told me to eat only two slices of bread for the second meal.
- Add one Mozzarella Ball of white cheese, which is about 125 grams of Mozzarella Light, 6 cm of cucumber, and five baby tomatoes.
- You can put one slice of ham on each slice of bread. Just two slices of ham for my second meal is a compromise. After all, ham is not that bad as sausages.
- You may add one teaspoon of Extra Virgin oil to your tomatoes and add a little bit of black pepper for taste.

Third Meal

- Take a small piece of boiled chicken without skin, boiled potatoes or boiled brown rice, tomato dressing with Greek yogurt and tomato concentrate.
- You may add a small piece of onion and garlic, fried with Extra Virgin oil, to your tomato dressing.
- Preferably pair this with an Italian green salad with a little bit of Extra Virgin oil and one teaspoon of honey, and squeeze a little amount of lemon into your salad.

Fourth Meal

It could be something like your second meal.

For Drinks

- Green tea with dried roses or bits of dried prickly pear.
- Green tea with dried lemon or whatever provides a flavor that is indispensable for getting rid of sugar.

Green tea is sweet, contains no calories, and is vegan and natural. The idea of green tea is to reduce sugar cravings. Sugar should be eliminated completely for healthy weight loss. Instead of sugar, you can use natural sweeteners like Erythritol / Erytrytol, or Erythrit/, which has all zero calories.

- At least 2 liters of Mineral Still Water daily is strongly advisable to stay hydrated.

The diet above was prescribed to me by my dietician. In the above example diet, you may have noticed that we have eliminated animal fat, sugar, and sausages (they are processed, and it is not a good idea to eat processed foods. I used to love grilled sausages, but to make healthy changes to your daily diet; you should exclude processed foods), cakes, sweets, and chocolates.

The above-mentioned meals should give you an idea of what to eat. However, we are all of different sizes, so we have to know how many calories we need to just make our meal consumption satisfy our needs without activities. If we have physical activity, we should multiply the above kcalories by 1.4 or 1.5. The result of such calculations represents the calories our body needs to function. For example, if I wanted to walk along a distance of 3 km, I used to add a banana and a sandwich to my diet.

I religiously cooperate with my dietician. It motivates me to impress her. I have consultations with her, and if I have no results, it would be a shame to me and a bad reference for her. Yet, not any more, it looks that my dietician has become so popular that I have to book a visit with her at least one week in advance and I go to her once a week. That is why I have to be serious and consistent in my journey. I am very tall, and now, having gone down to 123.6 kg, I seem to look more attractive than before. As someone who used to be fit until their late 50s and then suddenly had to face the reality of obesity with hypertension, seeing my weight loss progress has upped my confidence.

When I am somewhere in public and walk by some places that have huge mirrors, my reflection makes me feel happy about myself. It is not just about how I look; it is about how I feel. I feel proud of the steps I have taken and continue to take. Just yesterday, I bought a Barcelona football T-shirt, and today, I put it on and looked at myself in the mirror. And you know what I saw? I saw a Spanish footballer. This T-shirt is a little larger, so it perfectly covers my not-too-large belly. This reflection is like a reward for me. We should reward ourselves with an elegant appearance and hide imperfections if that is what makes us happier about ourselves- there is no shame in that, regardless of what others tell us. However, I am not suggesting to hide your pounds instead of sheading them.

My goal is to have 115 kg. Obtaining the targeted weight does not mean that I can start eating like when I was 30, unhealthy and unfiltered. Of course, we can make occasional exceptions after getting the results, yet we must not go back to old habits.

I wrote that the diet shown above is an example diet. It means that it was written for an obese person of 192 cm in height and 131.5 kg in weight without any physical activity.

However, keeping in mind the kcalories, this diet can be adopted by anyone. I purposely wrote it shortly to keep it simple. It is easier to explain dieting by having a simplified version of all those factors you have to analyze to understand crucial mechanisms.

Key:

- If you want to reduce your weight, you have to take away 400 kilocalories from kilocalorie intake you need to maintain your weight (which was 2400 in my case).

- During losing weight, you may have to take vitamin D3 4000 units daily and good tablets with omega 3 from salmon oil – 2 capsules daily. This is for an adult person.

- You cannot estimate the precise amount of kcalories your body needs, and you cannot assess the products you use in terms of kcalories for your daily consumption precisely.

- You have to use a scale and measure, e.g., chest, belly, waist, and below. Jot down your data and the food you eat. And finally, draw conclusions to correct the amount of your food intake.

- What I wrote above is true. Yet, you can also try to assess calories you need right now to maintain even your obese body by noting amounts of food you eat during a day.

- Once knowing how much kcalories your body needs, you can adjust healthy meals targeting the calories after taking away 400 kcalories, to have a proper calorie deficit to lose weight.

How to assess calories:

- Each product you buy contains ingredients with kcal and/or grams.

- My dietician told me to have only 3 slices of bread and 4 large potatoes or 7 small potatoes for dinner

- You should have a kitchen scale. Traditional one is very simple. Whatever you put on it, it shows how much it weights. I love electronic kitchen scales. You can juggle with useful simple features. There are usually two buttons: one is AN/TARA and the other is MODE. This scale costs 7.5 US dollars. Cheap and precise.

Mode is to choose units: grams, lb:oz /imperial units/ or ml of milk /milliliters of milk/.

AN/TARA is to tell the display to show zero whatever is or is not on the scale.

EXAMPLES:

You want to know how much oat flakes there are in a cup. By MODE choose grams. Put on scale a cup. It shows how much a cup weights in grams. By pressing AN/TARA the scale shows 0. You are slowly adding oat flakes into the cup until it shows 30 grams. Now, you have 30 grams of oat flakes. Your scale does not show the weight of a cup, despite the cup is not the scale.

You want to know how much HUMUS is on your spoon. Put the whole package of HUMUS on scale. Mode is set to grams. You press AN/TARA and it shows 0 grams. You take a spoon of HUMUS from the package, and the scale shows -5 grams.

This scale is logical. It shows: 0-5grams=-5grams.

I know that there are so many details here. Yet, after some time you will use your clean hands, spoons and you will just prepare dishes without using scales like a robot.

Final thing:

-Some people can use EXCELL where you can include a "library" of different ingredients and while writing your meals consisting of different ingredients input in grams,Excell will sum it up and show kcal of all meals throughout a day,

-Fitatu Premium like 10$ per year on your smartphone. You can choose ready meals or modify them to have a meal of your choice showing all kcal.

You can have enumerated meals throughout your day and throughout weeks and months

-you can buy your own scale for measuring your weight. Prices vary. The cheapest one is about 30 $. For 500$ you can buy a scale measuring not only the total weight, but fat, fluids and muscles.

Chapter 6: Losing Weight, the Healthy Way II

I am a 61-year-old individual who has been facing obesity in my life, have had many accompanying medical problems, including heart problems, hypertension, and more, and have managed to regain health and proper weight. Therefore, you already know that whatever I write is based on, or at least verified, by my own experience. If you write a book after only reading multiple others without having faced your own personal challenge in your life, then that piece of writing loses its credibility. You have to prove that what you are advising and advertising actually works.

Let me give you an example from the story of Bruce Lee. He wrote his book about martial arts, was at the promotion of his book, and at the same time had just recovered from serious medical treatment. Somebody demanded that he should prove his martial techniques work without considering his medical condition. Nevertheless, Bruce Lee took the challenge and won. It was brutal, but life is brutal.

Therefore, I state that if you dare to advise me what to do, and you do not have your personal experience to support it, I would just not believe you. And I believe that would be the case for you as well. To spice it up, I state that doctors are not perfect. I often seek for a second opinion from a second doctor.

Let me give you one more example from the movie "Walk the Line" about Johnny Cash. Before enjoying his career, Johnny tried to record his song and went through an audition. His songs were about God, yet his singing could not convince a listener, so this song was rejected. Therefore, you have to sound convincing to others with your story to be accepted.

I repeat one more time: You must have personal experiences to support your expression to sound credible. I state that whatever I write about healthy lifestyle is based on my personal experience backed up by knowledge of doctors and books. What is more, my writing about healthy food and lifestyle changes includes background medical problems and the necessity to introduce physical activity to enable me to enjoy good weight, health, and happiness in my life. This is why I picked up my pen and all the words I have: for you. For you to gain inspiration and for you to change what needed to be changed.

You must realize that hard work and dedication to achieve your goals will make you appreciate your achievements more. On the contrary, if something comes easy, you won't even notice what you should enjoy.

This is why I implore you to reorganize the way you look at a healthy-life journey before you start walking down one. You won't eat a salad one day and wake up the next feeling like you lost five pounds; this is not how weight loss works. You will find many "Lose Weight in 15 days" and "Get Slim in a Week" blogs and videos online, and let me just tell you: they are only scams taking advantage of your desperation to look and feel better. These shortcuts may promise rapid results with minimal effort, but nothing that compromises your well-being can be healthy, for sure? Because that is what they do. These shortcuts are not healthy. You may lose weight but at what cost? Your electrolytes may go haywire, your immune system may get weak, and your mental health may also suffer.

These quick fixes and even healthy dieting often leave out important nutrients your body needs to stay healthy. When you drastically cut calories or skip entire food groups, you're missing out on essential vitamins and minerals. This can make you feel tired, weak, and even sick. Then there's the problem with your metabolism, which is like your body's engine. When you go on a super strict diet, your body thinks it's not getting enough food, so it slows down your metabolism to conserve energy. This might help you lose weight at first, but it can make it easier to gain it back later on.

Quick fixes can also mess with your head. They can make you feel bad about yourself and lead to unhealthy thoughts about food. And when you lose weight quickly and then gain it back just as fast, (like a boomerang, as I often say), it can make you feel even worse.

Chapter 5: Why Quick Fixes Aren't the Answer

Let's talk about those tempting shortcuts promising fast weight loss. You know, the crash diets, extreme cleanses, or magic pills that claim to melt away pounds in no time. While they might seem like a quick fix, they actually come with some serious risks.

These quick fixes often leave out important nutrients your body needs to stay healthy. When you drastically cut calories or skip entire food groups, you're missing out on essential vitamins and minerals. This can make you feel tired, weak, and even sick.

Quick fixes work due to a certain component /e.g. a magic pill/, which is tremendously unhealthy in the first place.

Quick fixes can also mess with your head. They can make you feel bad about yourself and lead to unhealthy thoughts about food. And when you lose weight quickly and then gain it back just as fast (which often happens), it can make you feel even worse. Here is the thing: those quick fixes rarely lead to long-term success. Sure, you might drop a few pounds fast, but chances are you'll gain them back once you stop the diet. It's like a never-ending cycle of losing and gaining weight, which can be super frustrating and demoralizing especially losing and gaining back will make you weaker with each such a cycle.

So, instead of falling for the promise of a quick fix, it's better to take a slow and steady approach to weight loss. Focus on eating balanced meals, staying active, and making healthy choices every day. It might take longer, but the results will be worth it in the end – and you'll feel better both physically and mentally.

Remember, there's no shortcut to true health and happiness!

Now, this begs the question: what about supplements? Since the crash diets, extreme cleanses, and magic pills that promise to fix you are out of the way, can you improve your health with supplements?

As someone who has made use of them to get their health back on track after facing obesity and weight gain issues, I would say: Yes.

Although getting exposed to the world of supplements can be confusing as there are many such products and obviously you cannot buy all of them from Vitamin A to Zinc. But don't worry, I will take you through the role of dietary supplements in your daily life, amongst other things. I believe that you need to research everything you put inside your body, and supplements are one of them.

Let us look at a definition of a supplement. A supplement is a product that is intended to supplement or enhance the diet by providing vitamins, minerals, herbs, amino-acids or other dietary ingredients. They are to fill nutritional gaps especially while dieting, or aging. To me, a magic pill from an internet is not a supplement. All those quick-fixes advertised on internet are posing a serious threat to our health. If they were safe, and properly tested, they would end up in a pharmacy.

Supplements can be a valuable tool for healthy weight management, but it's crucial to understand their limitations. They are not replacements for a healthy diet. A balanced diet rich in fruits, vegetables, whole grains, and lean protein should be the foundation of your health and weight management efforts. Healthy dieting, healthy eating habits, and consistency should be your go-to for achieving your weight goals.

Supplements play a supportive role by:

- **Filling Nutrient Gaps:** If your diet lacks essential vitamins and minerals due to restrictive eating habits, picky eating, or certain medical conditions, supplements can help bridge those gaps and ensure you get the required nutrients for your best health.

- **Supporting Specific Needs:** Certain supplements might be beneficial for individuals with specific needs. For example, athletes may require additional protein or electrolytes because they are losing so many calories and water.

- **Enhancing Specific Functions:** Some supplements, like fiber or green tea extract, may offer modest benefits for specific functions. Fiber can make you feel full and regulate digestion, while green tea extract might slightly increase metabolism.

A healthy diet should be your primary focus. If, however, you wish to add supplements for a healthier lifestyle, you need to be mindful of choosing the right one. With countless supplements available, choosing the right ones can be overwhelming. Here are some key factors you need to look for:

- **Scientific Evidence:** Look for supplements backed by reliable scientific evidence demonstrating their effectiveness for your desired purpose. Don't be swayed by marketing claims that sound too good to be true.

- **Ingredient Quality:** Go for reputable brands that use high-quality, well-researched ingredients. Third-party certifications like USP (United States Pharmacopeia) or NSF International (NSF) indicate independent testing for purity and potency.

- **Dosage Matters:** Always follow the recommended dosage on the label. Exceeding the recommended dosage can be harmful and can be counter- effective.

- **Potential Interactions:** Supplements can interact with medications you're taking. Consult your doctor or dietician before starting any supplements to avoid potential complications. While aging like even over 40 or 50, you tend to take more supplements or prescribed medication, so be more cautious for possible interactions.

Don't go for magic pills that promote quick fixes. Yes, you may find yourself desperate to achieve results as soon as possible, and you may feel like going for the "Lose weight in 10 days" magic pills will help you with just that, but in cases like this, sustainable weight loss will always be a challenge. Sustainable weight loss and optimal health require long-term lifestyle changes, not a magic pill. So be wary of supplements promising rapid weight loss or dramatic improvements in health. What is more, I browse social media and I am noticing things. Of course, there are lots of magic pills. Those pills you can buy by contacting a dealer. They will send it to you through UPS or many other ways. The thing is that even my cardiologist made me aware of a simple truth. All those pills and other things you buy from a pharmacist are after proper testing and usually are more reliable. Whereas, whatever you buy over internet is usually without conducting proper tests. Over internet, you can buy medication for injections to lose weight. You are choosing an option how much kilograms you want to lose. A certain nurse told me that these injections cause complications. And one more thing, You can have your body to be modelled by special laser machines getting rid of fat. **My rhetorical question for you is: Is it safe? I am 100% sure that at least it is not neutral to our body!!!!!!!!!!!!!!!!**

I must admit that I tried to order sth. from internet. The dealer knew my number and phoned me after a long time. You are in their database and they will call you from time to time. There is more to it. It is not how I have been brought up, but in such situations just disconnect.

The next thing you need to look out for are testimonials and celebrity endorsements. Personal anecdotes and celebrity endorsements are not reliable scientific evidence. First of all, celebrities get paid to promote things; they don't do it for free. You have no idea whether they work or not or are healthy or not, so don't just blindly buy a magic pill because you saw your favorite actress posting about it on Instagram.

Next, don't be fooled by complex-sounding ingredients. Many products include ingredients made fancy by jargon, and people buy them after being impressed by reading them. **Research the components of a product and understand their purpose. Always read a product leaflet provided with the product or medication.**

Some other supplement-related advice I can give you is to keep an eye on magnesium. While some minerals like magnesium are essential for health, it's important to note that even correct doses can contribute to kidney stones in certain individuals. Consult your dietician before taking magnesium supplements, especially if you have a history of kidney stones.

Next on the list is Diuretics. Diuretics are medications that increase urine output and can help remove excess fluid from the body by drinking at least 2 liters of still mineral water, and at the same time, they can help lower blood pressure for those who have hypertension issues, as I do. However, it's important to be aware of their limitations. Although, they don't directly target fat loss; diuretics help remove excess fluids from your body. They can lead to electrolyte imbalances by depleting electrolytes, particularly potassium. Which is why taking potassium supplements may be the way to go. Scientists so far have not discovered diuretics to get rid of sodium only responsible for hypertension. As in such a case, it would be perfect.

Supplementation is often necessary to counteract diuretic-induced potassium loss. Potassium is a vital electrolyte for muscle function, nerve transmission, and maintaining healthy blood pressure. To manage potassium in your body, increase your intake of potassium-rich foods like bananas, avocados, leafy greens, and potatoes. If needed, your doctor may recommend potassium supplements, but be cautious of overdoing it. Just take one tablet of potassium a day, and give blood samples every 4 months for analysis if you take diuretics.

Before you go on with taking supplements, however, I would advise you to take guidance from a healthcare professional first esp. if for you all supplements look indispensable and you just are ready to buy them from A to Zinc. Like for me, I have my dietician by my side, and she provides me with invaluable guidance by assessing my specific needs, evaluating my dietary habits, and identifying my potential nutrient deficiencies. Based on your health profile and objectives, they can recommend suitable supplements and appropriate dosages, though appropriate dosages are on the leaflet inside the package of a supplement and especially a medication with all important info and side-effects. If they provide you with such a leaflet, it is for the reason. You should read it. You cannot say that you were not properly informed and can file a lawsuit. Furthermore, healthcare professionals can monitor your progress over time and make necessary adjustments to your supplement regimen as needed, ensuring your good health outcomes.

From my experience, I can tell you one thing for sure: Dietary supplements can be a valuable addition to a healthy lifestyle, but they shouldn't replace a balanced diet and healthy habits. Focus on getting most of your nutrients from whole foods and prioritize evidence-based supplements with guidance from a healthcare professional.

There is one more thing. After 40 or 50, you must realize that you are aging, so your body is not always capable of intaking all minerals and supplements from a balanced and healthy diet. We need vitamins, minerals and other supplements. And probably, we should not take them on and on, as our body can lose the ability to intake them from what we eat. Remember, a healthy and sustainable approach is key to achieving your weight loss and overall health goals. Whereas, whatever is sold by internet not from reputable companies is not safe at all. Those guys, who sell stuff over internet, they are anonymous. You know only their mobile number, and products they sell may not be verified, and surely is not. Generally, supplements and medication in a pharmacy are quite safe. You have to read an attached leaflet carefully and if you do not understand sth. ask a pharmacist for an information. Usually, vitamins and minerals are safe if you take usually one tablet a day, or in some cases two. I do not know about possible interactions, or side-effects in case of vitamins and minerals. I know that magnesium can help in creation of kidney stones. Yet, even an ordinary salt is no good for hypertension. Salt can be bought in a shop. If you look at my simplified definition of supplements, supplements are not only minerals and vitamins. Yet, they are not magic pills sold over the internet. From what I write, you may have an impression that I have my cardiologist at my side with tandem of my dietician.   The truth is they are at my disposal privately. Even if I am insured, I have to pay for my cardiologist and my dietician. Idealistically, I have my family doctor at my disposal. She should direct me to a cardiologist and to a dietician, and I should not pay. Of course, she will, yet for a specialist doctor's visit, you have to wait months, or one year maybe. That is why if I know that I have heart problems, and I need to go to a cardiologist privately, I do not need a filled paper from my family doctor. I just contact a private cardiologist. If I am over weighted, I go to a dietician. A private one.

To sum it up, I go to my cardiologist once a year for scanning of my heart and in case of emergency. All medication from my cardiologist can be prescribed by my family doctor if they are in her computer system. Monitoring my blood pressure I do by myself and have to make sure that I take medication according to my cardiologist's instruction.

Actually, after nearly one year of going to my dietician, I may just thank her for all the work, cos she educated me about most of things I should know. Although, she does not charge me much, I am not rich enough not to see limiting expenses.

Taking into consideration, that I noticed positive correlation between being slimmer and not having hypertension, I am interested to have a proper weight and I pay attention to what I eat and drink. That is the reason, I share my story.

In News I hear that there are more and more even obese children even in a primary school. Not only them, they are less skillful even while throwing a ball. And I do not even mean scoring a basket with a ball. Actually, I notice obese people on the street, and especially seeing them eating a large pizza or eating a large PLATE OF ICE-CREAM, I am just asking myself a question: "Do they not realize what they are doing?". 20 or 30 years ago, it was different. In my country, for some time during communism we had cards with limitation how much meat we could buy. It was rationalized. Yet, people at that time were slim. At physical education 46 years ago, we had to do such elaborate jumps, and all other exercises, that it was nearly like in a Circus. I am not joking.

All in all, my example and what I see proves the point that we have to keep balance in everything. We have to keep in mind that political correctness should not allow to say that sb. is fat. I understand it. Yet, obesity is not only looks. It is also unhealthy. This book is not about being kind and paying complements. It is about life. It is about how to survive in this more and more complicated world, where actually in some cases like retirement a human being is like a product. It is all about business. Whereas, I do not perceive others as products. Left-overs from our table land in my garden, where animals like: birds, a cat, dogs, squirrels thrive. They are our companions. Actually, they are our only companions. People nowadays are busy and do not have time to talk longer than 3 minutes a few times during a year.

Chapter 7: The Heart and the Health

The heart. Oh, the heart. This organ is everything inside your body. It makes your body. It makes you. Without it, we are nothing. It is the heart that stops when you take your last breath. The brain stays working after you die for some time, but it is the heart, the flat-line sound, that determines whether you are here or gone. So, the heart should be your most precious in your body, no?

We take many things for granted in life, and our body is one of them. If we are born healthy due to the bounty of the higher forces, we continue with our lives and don't express our gratitude for being healthy until that one moment of shift arrives, that one moment that opens our eyes. For me, that moment would be the hospital, I suppose. You don't realize the good things you had until something crashes- a bubble if you live in one.

Finding out I had hypertension was one of the hardest times of my life. I was told, then, that my artery was so big that a heart operation would soon follow. Imagine being told that; imagine my helplessness as I realized that my heart might fail me enough to need to be operated on. So, yes, well, it was not an easy time, but I pulled through. For four years, I took my medicine, I focused on myself, and I pulled through so well that I haven't taken my hypertension pills for two months now! If that doesn't scream progress, well, I don't know what will.

Obesity and hypertension are known allies. Obesity can cause hypertension or worsen it if you have it. While both may be allies, they are both your biggest enemies. So, while sitting on the hospital bed, so weak that my blessed father had to help dress me up, all I thought was, I have to fight both of them. Of course, winning altogether is the hardest because getting rid of a health issue completely is by far the most challenging battle of all. It requires persistence beyond what you can imagine. So, while leaving them behind completely would be the ultimate goal, in battles of health, you first win by trying. You try your hardest to regain control of your health and your life along with it.

Right now, at 61, I have lost a lot of weight, and my heart problems are getting lesser and lesser as compared to all that time. But to reach this point, I had to shift the way I thought and acted. I had to transform myself into a wielder of change for my own self. You ask why it was important? For those who are not that deeply aware of hypertension, blood pressure is the force exerted by circulating blood against the walls of blood vessels. It is essential for delivering oxygen and nutrients to tissues throughout the body. However, consistently high blood pressure, known as hypertension, can increase the risk of serious health complications, including heart disease, stroke, and kidney damage. And when you have obesity as well, that adds up the risks of worsening hypertension, diabetes, breathing problems, arthritis, and whatnot. So you can see the pickle I was in? The threats to my health, well-being, and quality of living were graver. Something had got to give.

When you have both obesity and hypertension, the primary goal is always to work on your weight, and so did my doctor and dietician. While I was on medications, my focus was on reducing my weight because that is how you kill two birds with one stone. This is how diet became the most crucial part of my journey.

Diet serves as a cornerstone in the management of both obesity and hypertension, offering a powerful tool for achieving and maintaining optimal health. By understanding the intricate relationship among dietary choices, body weight, and blood pressure regulation, individuals can make informed decisions to support their journey toward improved well-being.

The modern diet that has now become a part of every average person's life, like the high intake of processed foods, saturated fats, and added sugars, has been closely linked to the obesity epidemic. These dietary patterns are sure to make you exceed your recommended calorie intake to maintain your weight and, at the same time, promote weight gain and adipose tissue accumulation, increasing the risk of obesity-related complications like hypertension.

But you shift around to a healthy, well-balanced diet that prioritizes whole, nutrient-dense foods, and you can achieve and maintain a healthy weight. By making fruits, vegetables, whole grains, lean proteins, and healthy fats a necessary part of your meals, you can fuel your body with the essential nutrients needed to function the best while keeping your calorie intake in check.

The choices you make for your diet will undoubtedly influence body weight. And because of the control of your body weight, it will play a direct role in blood pressure regulation.

At this point, I would like to bring in the role of potassium and sodium in hypertension as well. High-sodium diets, commonly found in processed and restaurant-prepared foods, can lead to fluid retention and increased blood volume, which in turn raises blood pressure levels. In contrast, diets rich in potassium, magnesium, and fiber have been associated with lower blood pressure and reduced risk of hypertension. Potassium helps to counteract the effects of sodium by promoting the excretion of excess fluid and relaxing blood vessel walls, so taking potassium supplements works for the best.

While a healthy diet that I have shared in previous pages stays in place, there are some considerations that those with hypertension have to make specifically:

1. **Sodium Reduction:** Limiting sodium intake is crucial for hypertension management. You should aim to consume less than 2,300 milligrams of sodium per day, or even less if you have hypertension or are at risk. This involves reducing the consumption of processed foods, canned soups, salty snacks, and fast food and going for fresh, whole foods prepared at home.

2. **Potassium:** Potassium plays a key role in fluid balance and blood pressure regulation. Foods such as bananas, oranges, spinach, sweet potatoes, and avocados are excellent sources of potassium and should be incorporated into the diet regularly to support hypertension management. To assist in high potassium levels, taking potassium supplements will also help combat the threats of excess fluid.

3. **Lean Proteins:** Choosing lean protein sources such as poultry, fish, legumes, and tofu over high-fat meats can help reduce calorie intake and support weight management efforts. These protein sources are also rich in nutrients like magnesium, which has been linked to lower blood pressure levels.

4. **Whole Grains and Fiber:** Whole grains, such as brown rice, quinoa, oats, and whole wheat bread, are rich in fiber and other essential nutrients that promote satiety and digestive health. Fiber has been shown to help regulate blood sugar levels and cholesterol levels, both of which are important factors in hypertension management.

5. **Healthy Fats:** Incorporating sources of healthy fats, such as olive oil, nuts, seeds, and fatty fish like salmon and mackerel, can help improve heart health and reduce inflammation. These fats provide essential omega-3 fatty acids, which have been associated with lower blood pressure and a reduced risk of cardiovascular disease.

I want you to know one thing, though. This guideline is just general for a person with hypertension, but a lot rides on what your doctor says. When you are at a crucial enough stage that you are at risk of an operation, like I was, you can't make huge changes to your lifestyle without having talked to your doctor or dietician first.

What I know is not through intuition but from the assistance of a young, knowledgeable, and ambitious dietician with a Master's degree. She is equipped with a special scale that is connected to a computer. When you use this scale, a small electrical current flows through your body from your bare feet and hands. Resistance of excess fluid, muscles, and grease is different. Smart software can analyze changes in electrical current and assess the amount of grease, fluids, and muscles. Such a scale is worth even 3000 US dollars. There are decent scales for 500 dollars. The cheapest scale costs only 50 dollars, but it shows only the total weight and is not so precise if you wish to know the details of your condition- which helps, trust me!

Regular monitoring of blood pressure levels is a must for managing hypertension and preventing complications. So, you need to work closely with your healthcare provider like I do. I know from experience that they are the best people to develop a personalized treatment plan that includes regular blood pressure checks, medication management, and lifestyle interventions for you to be in your best health. If you remain proactive about scheduling regular check-ups and following up with your healthcare team as needed, I am sure your blood pressure control and overall health will see huge amounts of progress.

And while we are still on the topic of overcoming hypertension, I want you to know that we have discussed only one end of the spectrum: dietary change. Diet, I would say, is the biggest factor when it comes to your weight control, but is that the only thing? How else do you stay healthy? What more can you do? Because when you start this journey of healthy life, you can't just control what goes in your mouth and exercise until you sweat and then call it a day. It is called a lifestyle change for a reason, so it means you have to unlearn all your habits and start anew. It sounds scary? It is not. At all. If you believe you can do anything, remember, you can do anything. And if your hypertension is not in a good place, you have got to give it your all, my friend. Yes, it will be overwhelming; all changes and big shifts in life are. But one step at a time, and suddenly, you will have walked a mile.

So, while you continue to eat healthy, also focus on your physical activity. Exercise is a must, I repeat, a must, for maintaining a healthy weight, improving cardiovascular fitness, and lowering blood pressure. Aim for at least 150 minutes of moderate-intensity aerobic activity or 75 minutes of vigorous-intensity activity each week, along with muscle-strengthening activities on two or more days per week. In your workout routine, add the activities you enjoy, such as walking, swimming, cycling, or dancing, and strive for consistency in your exercise routine.

I have mentioned this before as well, but I am really taken with running. Have been for years. I even ran half a marathon. And what other pleasure does it give me than make me aware of my own strength? I think that is the biggest gift that continuous physical activity can give you: your awareness of what you are capable of doing. Don't take physical activity as a chore when it is just you pushing yourself to be better. But whatever you do, don't take on stress!

Hypertension and stress are also good old pals too. Chronic stress can contribute to elevated blood pressure levels and increase the risk of heart disease. If you practice stress-reduction techniques like mindfulness meditation, deep breathing exercises, yoga, tai chi, or progressive muscle relaxation, you can lower your stress hormones and promote relaxation.

I have seen many people resort to alcohol or smoking as a way to lower their stress and have distractions, but those are the last things you should do when you want to get healthy. You want to know what having alcohol and smoking is like when you have obesity and hypertension? Like walking in a shark's den with blood all over your body.

Excessive alcohol consumption can raise blood pressure and make you gain weight, among other health issues. For a healthy heart, you will need to let go of that beer. And the tequila. And the wine... you get my point. Limit alcohol intake to moderate levels, defined as up to one drink per day for women and up to two drinks per day for men, and that too if you really really have to. Or else, just don't have it. You can try juices, mocktails, and other non-alcoholic beverages to satisfy your thirst.

As for smoking, I am sure there is not much to say. There is a reason why your TV and radio don't have cigarette ads. It is a major risk factor for hypertension and cardiovascular disease. If you like having a puff, do yourself a favor and quit smoking, for that is one of the most important steps you can take to improve your overall health and reduce your risk of heart disease.

Instead of walking towards these harmful substances as distraction, look for healthy outlets for stress, always, such as engaging in hobbies, spending time in nature, or connecting with loved ones. Many people don't pay heed to this, but your physical and mental health walk side by side. You get worse in the head, and your body will realize it.

Give your mind a break, even when it feels hard. Rest your mind with your body as well. And well, just rest! Just because you are on this healthy lifestyle journey does not mean you have to do something every hour of every day; that is absurd! Your body needs plenty of time to breathe in peace. Or better yet, sleep. Quality sleep is essential for overall health, including blood pressure regulation. Aim for 7-9 hours of uninterrupted sleep per night, and establish a regular sleep schedule to support your body's natural circadian rhythm.

I know that many people have trouble sleeping, so try to create a relaxing bedtime routine, avoid caffeine and electronic devices before bedtime, and create a comfortable sleep environment to promote restful sleep. I am sure sleep will find you soon enough.

By incorporating these healthy lifestyle changes into your routine, along with dietary modifications, you can kick your hypertension to the curb. Or maybe not to the curb, but enough so that it doesn't stand over you. And when you do that, you can improve your cardiovascular health and enhance your overall well-being. Remember that small changes can lead to significant improvements over time, so focus on making sustainable lifestyle adjustments that support long-term health goals.

Chapter 8: Staying Active is Staying Healthy

As a 61-year-old man, I won't say that I have the spirit of the young anymore. And what I mean by that is I can't stay active and make myself sweat as much as an average young man fitter than me. I am limited by my age and my weight: I am aware. I am, perhaps, more aware because I have remained physically active for most of my life. I used to run a lot, cycle a lot, and move around a lot, so my body was very well accustomed to staying active and full of energy. But can I say the same for now? Probably not. Most of my transformation, about 80%, has been because of the 180-degree changes I have made to my daily diet. But do I wish I were more active? Absolutely yes. I cannot deny the benefits of staying active and moving your body, and neither should you.

Close your eyes and feel your body for a moment. You have joints at all the right places; have you thought about that? Your elbows to move your arms, your knees to move your legs… your body is meant to move in whatever capacity it can. So why would you want to stay in bed like a lazy couch potato and do nothing? Move around more: a goal to look forward to!

I cannot stress enough how important physical activity is to manage both obesity and hypertension. A small routine can make a huge difference, especially when you have all the weight and heart issues like I do. Even though because of my age, I usually only rely on my personal trainer to keep my muscles active, I feel myself healthier because of it.

When your body is active, in whatever way you can let it be active, it does not only burn calories. There are so many health benefits that keeping yourself active can bring you, including feeling a healthy body and a healthy mind. For all those who have both obesity and hypertension, regular physical activity can be transformative and offer you a pathway to weight management, cardiovascular health, and enhanced quality of life. Let me list you a few ways that exercise can help you.

Enhance Metabolic Function:

Regular exercise boosts metabolism and increases the body's efficiency in utilizing energy and facilitating weight loss. With a combination of aerobic and resistance training, you can elevate your resting metabolic rate and see sustainable weight management over time.

Improve Cardiovascular Health:

The cardiovascular benefits of exercise are profound and encompass improvements in heart function, blood flow, and vascular health. By engaging in regular physical activity, you can reduce your risk of hypertension, heart disease, and stroke while enhancing the efficiency of your cardiovascular system.

Promote Mental Wellbeing:

Exercise is so helpful as an antidote to stress, anxiety, and depression and promotes the release of endorphins and neurotransmitters associated with positive mood and emotional resilience. When you keep regular exercise in your daily life, you will often experience enhanced mental clarity, reduced stress levels, and an overall sense of well-being.

 Foster Long-term Health Habits:

Beyond its immediate benefits, exercise cultivates sustainable health habits and lifestyle changes that extend far beyond the gym. By integrating regular physical activity into your daily routine, you can develop a sense of empowerment, agency, and self-efficacy in managing your health.

While staying active is monumental in transforming yourself and seeing success in this health journey, you should remember that one size does not fit all when it comes to exercise, particularly for those people with obesity and hypertension. So if you have either or both of those, you need to look after your needs first. For example, consider factors such as fitness level, medical history, and personal preferences.

For a customized workout routine- suited for you, consider having your fitness level, heart health, and any medical issues thoroughly evaluated. This may involve consulting doctors and potentially doing specialized fitness tests to establish a baseline. It's also key to remember to take things gradually. If you've been inactive, easing into more physical activity is crucial to avoid injury and keep you motivated. Begin with low to moderate-intensity exercises like walking or swimming. Then, over time, you can slowly increase how long, hard, and often you work out.

Also, another trip: embrace diversity! Embark on an exhilarating journey through various exercise modes. Combine heart-pumping aerobics, muscle sculpting re-sistance training, and flexibility-enhancing stretches. Spice up your routine with thrilling recreational sports! This vibrant mix keeps your workouts captivating, enjoyable, and supremely e-ffective.

But in your quest to become healthy no matter what, I will advise you to step back and chew only what you can take. Tune in to your body's whispers. Exercise demands attentiveness; heed signals of fatigue, discomfort, or pain. Adjust intensity or duration accordingly. Rest and recovery are vital components, allowing your body to rejuvenate and adapt to physical challenges.

People often seek assistance from trainers and doctors when creating their exercise plans. Even my present physical activity routine, no matter how extensive or lack thereof, is with the help of my trainer. These structured programs can guide you toward reaching health goals efficiently. Exercise specialists design regimens tailored to each individual's needs and abilities, providing a well-organized approach.

1. Aerobic Exercise:

Regular aerobic workouts form the core of any good fitness routine. Recommended activities like brisk walking, cycling, swimming laps, or doing aerobic dance- classes help improve cardiovascular health. They also burn calories and reduce hypertension risks for those struggling with obesity.

2. Resistance Training:

Complementing aerobic exercise, strength training builds muscle mass and boosts metabolism. By incorporating resistance exercises that target all major muscle groups, you can increase lean body weight. This improves overall body composition and enhances metabolic function, aiding fat loss.

3. Flexibility and Mobility:

Flexibility and mobility exercises are often overlooked but are crucial for maintaining joint health, preventing injuries, and improving overall functional capacity. Stretching, yoga, and Pilates are excellent options for promoting flexibility, balance, and range of motion.

4. Monitoring Progress:

Monitoring progress is essential for tracking improvements, adjusting exercise prescriptions, and maintaining motivation. This may involve tracking metrics such as weight, body composition, cardiovascular fitness, strength, and flexibility over time, providing valuable feedback on the efficacy of the exercise program.

But while I talk and blab and rant about all the health benefits of staying active to stay healthy, I am sure it won't fully register unless you have a full guide of what you can do. It is very easy to be vague and use fancy words to tell someone they need to change, but very few go deeper into the "how" of it all. From the start of this book, I have been real with you to help you, so if this has been overwhelming, let me give you my two cents.

For people with obesity and hypertension, the first step is mostly always to lose weight, and besides diet, starting a program of regular aerobic and muscle-strengthening exercises can work wonders to heal your body weight and your heart.

First, however, you need to get an assessment done. I wouldn't say this was a necessary step if you only wanted to stay active and had no underlying health problems. But when in cases of health issues like these, it is always best to have an opinion from an expert after they have evaluated your current fitness level, medical history, and risk factors.

Given your sedentary status according to your assessment, the exercise program will be designed to be progressive, starting with modest targets and gradually increasing over time. But from what I can tell you, generally, I would advise you to build up your physical activity targets over several weeks, starting with 10 to 20 minutes every other day to minimize potential muscle soreness and fatigue.

Your exercise program could incorporate a combination of aerobic exercise, resistance training, and flexibility exercises, again, according to your individual needs and preferences. Aerobic exercise, such as walking, may be the best part of your exercise program, and I am not saying that as someone who has a special affinity for running and walking. Walking helps you stay active without over-exerting yourself. It is just steps! One after another after another you go! You can supplement this by resistance training exercises targeting major muscle groups.

Throughout the program, regularly get your progress monitored to track improvements, adjust exercise prescriptions, and ensure safety and effectiveness. Progress metrics like heart rate monitoring, subjective ratings of perceived exertion, and periodic fitness assessments can help see how your body is responding to your physical activity regime. After each progress, you can make adjustments wherever you need them.

Through consistent participation in the exercise program, I am sure you can experience significant improvements in your cardiovascular fitness, muscular strength, weight management, and overall well-being. By gradually increasing the intensity and duration of your workouts and adhering to the principles of safe and effective exercise, you can achieve your health and fitness goals in no time.

Chapter 9: Avoiding Common Pitfalls

As I have identified before, the journey towards a healthier you and a healthier life is very tricky and very hard. You think you will take my advice from previous pages and be good to go? I wish I could tell you so. But that is not the case. You will stumble, and you will fall. Like I did many times. But at the end of the day, it is all about your determination to see things through.

In this winding path towards better health and sustainable weight loss, you will find many obstacles. Your cravings will be like the calls of the siren out in the city. Your resilience will feel like it is shattering. And that is only to name a few. But don't worry, for in this chapter, with my personal experience and insights; I will offer you a lantern to illuminate the pitfalls and a sturdy rope to help you climb out when you stumble.

There were many times when I craved something more, and when I say something more, I mean something yummy. Something that my heart would sing for but my body won't appreciate. Well, actually, with hypertension, my heart wouldn't either, but you get my point. Sometimes, the stomach just is not satisfied, and that is nothing to be alarmed about. It is normal. But at times like these, your diet can feel like torture. You may want to give everything up and just stuff your face in a bag of sodium-full chips. There may be a voice in your head telling you, "Just eat that cheese already." Now, this feeling is also normal. But you have to make sure you are not listening to that voice without any personal control. What do I mean by that?

I mean that you should allow yourself little indulgences from time to time. Given that you remain thoughtful of your portions. In fact, I would say it is good if you listen to that voice telling you the pizza will look yummier in your stomach rather than deprive yourself of it strictly. Strict diets are not sustainable; I know it. I know that you can focus on losing weight for three weeks with a strict miracle diet. You could lose even 15 kg. But that just won't work for the long term. After depriving yourself of all your cravings, you may eventually lose control. Say, after losing so much in 3 weeks, you may walk into Pizza Hut one day and eat and eat and eat for hours because you are hungry. And in doing that, you may gain like 4kgs overnight. If this cycle continues, you may eventually find yourself at your old weight in no time.

The thing is, the key to success is to introduce a healthy and low-caloric diet with few exceptions from time to time because we are human beings. Dieting should not be torture, so It is good to adapt slowly to different foods, even if we do not lose too much or nothing at all in the beginning.

However, that is not to say that you listen to your cravings all the time. That is the furthest thing from control. Cravings, like sly thieves in the night, can stealthily sabotage even the most disciplined of diets if you do not keep them under your thumb. You should be able to decide when to follow your cravings instead of your cravings, making you follow them. Understanding the triggers behind these insistent urges is the first step towards reclaiming control over your eating habits. Whether spurred by stress, boredom, or other emotional triggers, recognizing the root cause of your cravings empowers you to confront them head-on.

Cravings can be categorized into two main types: physiological and psychological. Physiological cravings are driven by biological factors such as nutrient deficiencies, hormonal fluctuations, or blood sugar imbalances. These cravings often manifest as specific urges for certain foods, such as chocolate cravings linked to magnesium deficiency or salty cravings indicative of sodium imbalances.

On the other hand, psychological cravings are rooted in our emotions, habits, and environmental cues. Stress, boredom, anxiety, and even social situations can trigger these cravings, leading us to seek comfort or distraction in food. Emotional eating, in particular, is a common response to negative emotions, as food provides a temporary escape from uncomfortable feelings. I believe this type of craving to be the worst because it just asks you to stuff your face without dealing with your feelings upfront. Far from the physical health aspect, cravings from all the emotional feelings are a way for your body to ask for temporary distractions, something that is only going to prolong your suffering. When you feel this way, it is better to take a moment for yourself, breathe in, assess your emotions, and then see what to do.

To effectively manage cravings, you may need to analyze where they are coming from. It's crucial to identify the triggers that set them off. What you could do is keep a journal to track your eating habits and note any patterns or correlations between your cravings and specific emotions, situations, or activities. Are you more likely to crave sweets when stressed? Do social gatherings trigger feelings of anxiety and subsequent overeating? By answering these questions for yourself, you can see your triggers and see what to do about them.

Once you know your personal triggers, you can develop strategies to combat cravings and break free from their grip. Mindfulness techniques, such as deep breathing or meditation, can help you tune into your body's signals and distinguish between true hunger and emotional hunger. Engaging in alternative activities, such as going for a walk, practicing a hobby, or calling a friend, can provide a healthy outlet for stress or boredom without resorting to food, which will ultimately jeopardize your progress if you listen to it without any caution.

Furthermore, incorporating a diverse range of nutrient-dense foods into your diet can help address physiological imbalances and reduce the frequency of cravings. Focus on building meals around whole foods rich in fiber, protein, healthy fats, and essential nutrients to promote fullness in your stomach and stabilize blood sugar levels. By nourishing your body with wholesome, nourishing foods, you can satisfy cravings at their root and cultivate a balanced approach to eating.

So, really, understanding the triggers behind cravings is the first step you can take to stay in control of your eating habits and have a healthier relationship with food.

That's the bit about cravings, but cravings usually occur out of nowhere, right? Like you would be lying in your bed and suddenly go "Damn, fries" in your head. But what do you do when the fries are in front of you, and all your family is munching on them in front of you while you have a carrot in your hand? That should be a form of torture, now, lol.

Social gatherings, with their yummy diet-free food and peer pressure, present a minefield for someone who is conscious of their diet. I understand that your friends and family don't have to follow and be considerate of your diet all the time, so what do you do?

I would say that before you go out, have a plan of action ready in your head. If you are going out to a restaurant, take stock of the event's menu in advance, if possible, and identify healthier options that align with your dietary goals. If attending a potluck or gathering at a friend's home, consider offering to bring a dish that meets your nutritional requirements so that there's at least one guilt-free option on the table that you can have.

I would also say that don't be afraid to communicate your dietary preferences and goals to the people who are hosting you or going out with you. Most people are accommodating and understanding, and if you just let them know that "Hey, I am on this journey of a healthier me," I am sure they would only motivate you along the way.

If you voice out your situation, you will not only make it easier for yourself, but also make people think about how there should be healthier options to be included in future gatherings to be able to include everyone. Additionally, sharing your journey with others may inspire and motivate them to make healthier choices as well.

Here is a tip: If you go to a buffet and see an array of options, go for lean protein sources, such as grilled chicken or shrimp, and load up on veggies and salads while exercising restraint with high-calorie, high-fat options. If indulging in alcoholic beverages, you can try lighter options like wine or spritzers. One thing I have said before and will say again: Be mindful of portion sizes! You don't want to stuff yourself by losing control. Without control, this journey is useless, trust me.

Another tip: Practice mindful eating techniques to fully savor and appreciate each bite, allowing yourself to indulge in moderation without overindulging. Take small, deliberate bites, chew slowly, and use all your senses to experience the flavors and textures of the food fully. By tuning into your body's hunger, you can avoid mindless munching and enjoy the social experience without sabotaging your progress.

Now that you have an idea about how you can go around the tricky maze of when to avoid unhealthy foods and when to not, let me just say that none of this will hold if you don't remain motivated on your journey. There will be countless moments when you may not want to go through with all of this.

One of the moments you may feel this way is with plateaus. Man, are those frustrating? But, well, I don't think escaping them is possible. My dietician told me it is normal, and I will tell you it is normal as well. If you don't know what they are, it is just when your body is not shedding any weight despite you working your hardest on it. Does that sound familiar now? And also annoying.

Consider plateaus a necessary stop you have to make. It's like when you are driving, and suddenly, the road becomes a circle. You are driving fast; your tires are okay, your car is okay, and everything is fine, but you are just not making any progress, seemingly. But that does not say anything about you doing anything wrong.

Why do these plateaus happen, you ask? It is when your body gets used to your exercise habits and your dieting habits. That doesn't sound too bad now, does it? Because your body has fully realized it is on the path to becoming healthy. I would say that is something to celebrate. But what do you do when this plateau is suddenly your reality? After all, you can't just give up on losing more weight if you still have health goals unchecked.

Change. That is one word, but also your answer. But before I scare you, this is only a little change. You go through big, big changes when you decide to become healthy. You cut curbs, you limit guilty food, you start to exercise, and on and on and on. But the good thing is that your body is already used to these big changes, so now you only have to make little ones. For example, you increase your physical exercise time by a few minutes. Or you can add in a few extra weights. Or you mix up your diet. There are so many ways!

In the end, it all comes down to how much you are willing to stick to this hard decision of becoming healthy. I know how I felt: it wasn't easy. It still is not easy. Some days are good, and you feel like you are strong, energized, and ready enough to take on the world. But then the reality of your health hits. I realize how my heart needs a lot more strength than I think, and this healthy lifestyle is too overwhelming. Like I say, it feels like a battle. Some days, you win, and some days, you are close to losing. But the key is to not lose. You have to believe in yourself because it is only if you believe that you will do.

I was working with my doctor and my dietician to lose all this weight and make healthy choices, so that was an immense help for me. I think support is most crucial when it comes to this health journey because when your own voice is failing, you, your friends, family, and advisors voice their motivations for you to continue.

So yes, the way I felt, and continue to feel, like I can't do this, you may too. And in times like these, you have to remember why you started in the first place. For me, I don't ever want to be weak enough to stick to the hospital bed. I have tried and tested it, and it sucks! I want to be able to walk on my own two feet, see the world with my own two eyes, and feel the energy in my beating heart. That is my truth, so I will continue to achieve it.

So, like this, in the crucible of adversity, resilience becomes your friend. It is this spirit that refuses to submit in the face of setbacks, the unwavering resolve that helps you to move on forward when the path ahead grows dim.

Epilogue

You know, when I started writing this book, I had only one aim in mind: to be a beacon of hope and inspiration. Does that sound cliché? Maybe it does; who am I to say? But that is what this hypertensive heart hoped for.

When I started my own health journey, I made it imperative for myself to pick up as many health books as possible to help me along the way. Because, of course, my wisdom back then in such topics wouldn't hold a candle against now. And while I found many good books that imparted great knowledge, I just couldn't find "the one." You know, "the one" book? The one that answers all the questions in your head without making you feel dumb? Some books, no matter how true, just don't explain stuff in the way a common man would be able to understand and resonate with, or at least that is something I felt.

Something else I felt: alone. I couldn't connect with the books I stumbled upon because they didn't feel personal. Sure, they must have been written based on the experiences and insights of professionals and experts, but I didn't feel heard. I didn't feel like I could truly feel the books I read in my heart. There were books with recipes, and I learned a lot from them. That is true, but sometimes, the meals were so sophisticated that going to the grocery to buy numerous items only to break your back trying to make it did not sit well with me. Making healthy meals should not test your patience or skills. It should be easy and hassle-free because you are not picking up ingredients to serve in a Michelin-star restaurant; you are using them to get to the healthy base of a dish you normally consume. Some books had too little information, and some books had too much to the point of you feeling cuckoo.

Why should getting healthy sound like a lecture in a medical school? It shouldn't. I felt like there was a need for something that could speak to people's souls, encourage them, and motivate them. And so I picked up my pen and my laptop, and voila. If, at times, you wondered, why should you even listen to me? After all, I am no doctor. I am no dietician. Who am I? In simple words, I am a voice on your right shoulder. I am the person holding your hand while you navigate your own health challenges.

Behind all these words I have written is a story I have been very open about. I have struggled, I have failed, I have overcome. I have gained insights that are so valuable that I can't just keep them to myself, but above all, I feel so motivated looking at my own progress that I don't see why others could not be or why you could not be. If out of a hundred people who picked this book up, I managed to motivate at least one, I would consider that a job well done.

This whole journey is an ongoing process. It is for me, and it will be for you. I just want you to know that you need to take a deep breath and just continue because I am continuing too. Am I at my optimum health? Hell no, I believe I have mountains to overcome, still. But the mountains I have already overcome, I am so proud of. You remember when I said I was so weak; how my father used to help me put on my undies? Compare that state of mine to now. I have worked hard and lost 8 kilograms of total weight and counting. I do not take Lapixen and Telmix Plus nearly at all. Two times per week, I take lapixen when my blood pressure is on the higher end, e.g. 127/96. But most of the time, it is about 120/80, which is a win, in my opinion.

Is mine a success story? I believe so. Success stories are not those that show unbeatable results; they are those that keep you moving with small wins every step of the way. And I want mine to reflect positively on you. You can do this, you have got this. Like I have. Let's continue to achieve our own milestones together. Like Arnold Schwarzenegger says: "ASTALA VISTA, BABY. I will be back!"

www.ingramcontent.com/pod-product-compliance
Lightning Source LLC
Chambersburg PA
CBHW051750250726
48659CB00001B/334